June 2012
To Bonnie,
For your
creative
herbal
home!

Tina Marie Wilcox

the creative herbal home

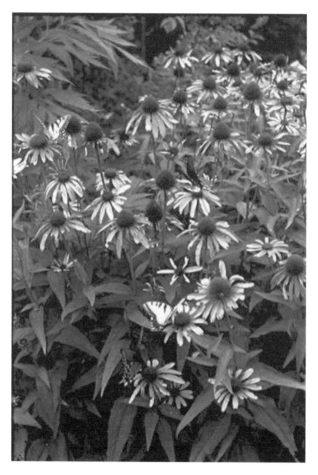

susan belsinger & tina marie wilcox

living with herbs series
herbspirit

Copyright Page

the creative herbal home
susan belsinger & tina marie wilcox © 2007

disclaimer:

photography, susan belsinger
authors' photo, steven foster
photo of tina marie in garden, ed schuh
printing layout, carrie camp
editing, sharon crain
indexing, lucie sargent
publisher, herbspirit, living with herbs series

text copyright 2007, susan belsinger & tina marie wilcox
photography copyright 2007, susan belsinger

creative printing & design
139 industrial park drive
hollister, mo 65672; 2nd printing, 2008

litho printers
904 west street
cassville, mo 65625; 3rd printing 2010

isbn # 0-9766771-1-3

dedication

this book is in honor of all of those herbalists
who have gone before us.
we are grateful for their fortitude, dedication, study,
their writing and keeping of records.
they are our inspiration.

we also dedicate this book to all of you herbies out there,
who share the love of the green plant spirits with us.
you are why we do what we do.
we create, garden, cook, teach, travel, research and write
with zeal and delight
so we can share all of these things
with like-minded individuals such as yourselves.

last but not least,
this book is for our youth who are the future,
with great hope that they will carry on
the love of cultivating plants,
protecting our environment
and creating awareness
to keep our mother earth
a healthy, sustainable and living planet.

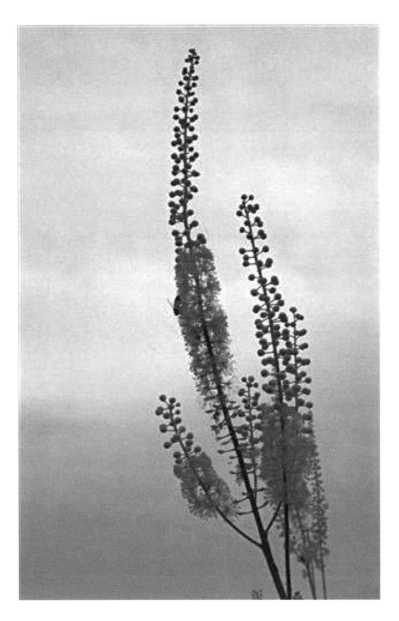

black cohosh flowers (Cimicifuga racemosa)

contents

acknowledgements

We give thanks to our families and friends who are always there for support. We are especially grateful to Sharon Crain for editing and to Lucie Sargent for preparing the index and catching typos.

Our sincere gratitude goes out to our extended herbal family—to all of our friends and colleagues with whom we grow our herbal knowledge and experiences.

Our appreciation for guidance, information and inspiration goes to our herbal and botanical gurus: Deni Bown, Francesco DeBaggio, Tom DeBaggio, Jim Duke, Steven Foster, Madalene Hill, Carl Hunter, Rosemary Gladstar, Jim Long, Rex Talbert, Billy Joe Tatum, Art Tucker and Elizabeth Warner.

These organizations share our love of herbs and friendship and make the world a better place: International Herb Association, Herb Society of America, The Committee of 100, United Plant Savers and the Women's Herbal Conference.

Thanks to the Herb Companion and Herbs for Health magazines and the staff at Ogden Publications for publishing our work—some of which is excerpted here.

To our creative, loving and productive women friends: Anne Abbott, Sherry Adaire, Audrey Belsinger, Sarah Clark, Kathryn Compton, Kathleen Connole, Pat Crocker, Becki Dahlstedt, Carolyn Dille, Gayle Engels, Cynthia Giss, Patricia French, Nanette Hatzes, Robin Johnsen, Pat Kenny, Susan Ketchum, Chloe Kirksey, Judy Klinkhammer, Bette Rae Miller, Leanna Potts, Deborah Redden, Marion Spear, Anne Thompson, and Cheryl Wilks; you have our heartfelt thanks.

introduction

Herbs are a way of life for us. Like you, we are distinctive individuals who are interested in using herbs to create beauty, happiness and health in our homes. We have written this book to share our methods for creatively using herbs in our homes everyday. Between the two of us, we have over fifty years of experience growing, buying and using herbs and essential oils.

Susan lives in a passive-solar home that she built with her husband, Tomaso, in Maryland between Washington D.C. and Baltimore. She grows herbs, flowers and vegetables on three acres of land in a rural setting; however, residing between two large East Coast cities her lifestyle is more cosmopolitan than that of Tina Marie.

Tina Marie lives on 28 acres of wooded mountaintop in north-central Arkansas in a small cabin. Her home is located a mile off the hardtop highway, far away from any city.

Although our lifestyles and households are very different, we share common household tasks. Cleaning and keeping our homes comfortable and free from pests provides on-going opportunities to experiment. Our bodies suffer much abuse as we work and play; we create ways to pamper ourselves and use our plants to support a healthy lifestyle.

The herbs in this book may be grown and gathered by our own hands or easily procured from the market or local shops. The essential oils, ingredients and equipment can be purchased from reputable local or online herbal businesses; see our **sources** in the back of this book.

Our chapter on **herbs** discusses the herbs that we use for preparations in this book. The chapter, **plant chemicals** is a decidedly scientific study. We believe that deeper knowledge empowers us to use herbs creatively and safely. Basically, we have endeavored to identify and explain scientific terms that we have found in herbal texts that have challenged us. The more that we know about the properties of the mediums we are working with, the more responsible and creative we can be.

Home is where the heart is and the heart of the home is in the kitchen. We gather in our kitchens to prepare delicious foods using culinary herbs to nourish our bodies. Herbal **infusions and decoctions** are simple, effective and basic to herbalism—*simples* were truly our first form of medicine. The kitchen is our laboratory for herbal alchemy where we create items for our pantry such as herbal vinegars and syrups, as well as our **household preparations** and remedies. Using the techniques in this book you too, can become a practicing home herbalist.

The **essential oils** (EOs) that we use most often are described and listed according to their attributes, along with appropriate cautions. We also prepare herbal creature comforts, cleaning aids and insect repellents. These are utilized to make our lives more comfortable in-and-around the house and are found in our chapters on **household preparations** and **gardening comforts**. Besides soothing and renewing the body, mind and spirit, you can create sensual pleasures for the bath and *boudoir* using recipes in our chapter on **body care**. We use our herbal remedies and recipes and **tinctures** for everything from keeping well and easing minor aches and pains, to boo-boos, colds and sniffles. In **herbal kits**, you will find instructions for putting together your own herbal home remedy kit and a travel kit as well.

Safety precautions are included. However, if you have health issues, a current malady, are taking prescription medications, are pregnant or nursing, consult your health care practitioner. Thoroughly research herbs, essential oils, and other ingredients, before using them. If you have questions or concerns, always use caution and safety. To make them easy for you to see, we have placed *cautions and warnings in italics* to set them off from the other text in this book (the only other italics that are used are for botanical nomenclature.) Cleanliness is of utmost importance. Keep your work area clean and use absolutely clean equipment, jars, utensils, etc. when preparing any of these recipes.

We are supportive of our environment and respect our earth; therefore, we recycle, grow our gardens organically and use organic, local, and/or the finest quality ingredients that we can find. Included is a chapter on **ingredients** that gives details about the best product to choose. For instance under oils, we discuss the different types and which ones are used for preparing massage or bath oils, making salves or for culinary use.

Also included are **definitions of terms** to familiarize you with words from macerate to menstruum and the difference between a distillate and hydrosol. We have provided a list of **sources** of our most-often used suppliers, businesses that we recommend, and a **bibliography** of our favorite books. We hope that this book will be a helpful companion as you make your own *creative herbal home*.

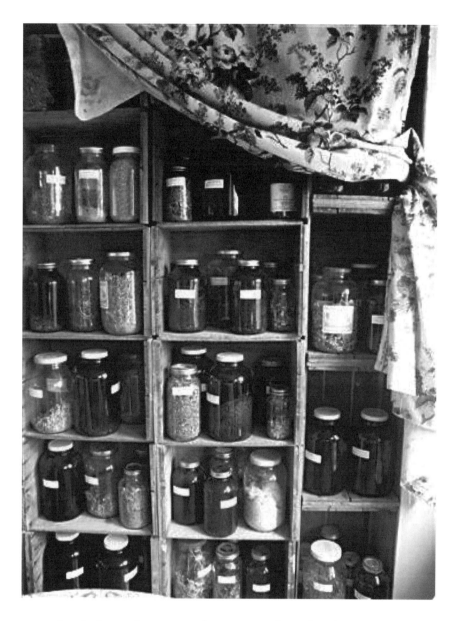

herbal apothecary at heartsong farm healing herbs

herbs

Every growing plant is useful to humanity for the oxygen it produces. Our nutrition, shelter, textiles, seasonings, therapeutic agents, fragrance, cleaning aids, comforts and addictions come directly or indirectly from the plant kingdom.

We grow our herbs, judiciously gather plants from our woods and pastures and buy fresh and dried botanicals. Herbs play important roles in our daily lives. By no means complete, the following list gives some insight into the properties of plants used in a creative herbal home. We hope that you will be inspired to continue your research into this fascinating and useful field of study.

In this chapter on herbs that we use, we give basic information. For those of you who have a background in herbs, we also include some science and scientific terms; so we can all broaden our understanding, as well as our herbal horizons. Critics of herbalism state that our confidence in the safety and efficacy of herbs is based on belief rather than hard data. We heartily agree that we do believe in the powerful therapeutic actions of plants. However, we respectfully disagree with the statement that our belief is not based on hard data. Published clinical trials and studies of the active constituents of plants abound in literature from all over the world.

The information given here is meant neither to prescribe nor to cure disease or injury. Please consult a medical practitioner if you have health issues. All plants are chemically complex (We are not responsible for the success or the problems incurred from your use or misuse of herbs.) When used, their actions may be gentle or quite alarming. Be sensible; perpetrate no harm and exercise personal responsibility for your actions.

preserving herbs

Like most other garden produce, herbs are best when they are fresh
and in season. In summer, they reach their peak of flavor and highest
concentration of essential oils. It is imperative to preserve this bounty
for the winter months when fresh herbs are not available to harvest.
Store the summer's harvest in your pantry, apothecary or freezer.
Enjoy the time spent preserving your herbs, knowing how glad you
will be to have their flavor and medicine all year.

harvesting herbs

Herbs should be harvested as the plants are forming their flower
buds, unless you want the flowers. You can rinse the plants with
water the day before harvest so that they will be as clean and dry as
possible at the time they are cut. Choose a sunny day and harvest
the herbs in the mid-morning, when their oils are strongest. Wait
until the morning dew has evaporated; it is best not to gather herbs
when they are wet. We give thanks to the plants and our mother
earth for providing us with herbal bounty as we harvest. Most
perennial and annual herbs can be harvested more than once a
season. Cutting them back about once a month during the summer
will encourage new growth and maximize your leaf harvest.

Cut perennials back to about one-third of their height. Cut annuals
just above the bottom set of leaves. Do not leave the cut herbs
out in the sun; take them into a shady area for sorting and tying
into bunches. If you live in a cold northern climate, do not prune
perennials too late in the fall, as this weakens the plants' resistance
to cold. The last harvest should be about 6 to 8 weeks before a hard
freeze so that the herbs have time to harden-off new growth.

For the last harvest of annuals, you can cut the tops and then pull up the roots. This way you are tidying up the garden for winter and reaping the harvest at the same time. If you have pulled whole plants, cut off the roots. Remove the brown bottom leaves and any spotted or bug-eaten ones. If the herbs are dirty, brush away the dirt. If you must wash them, rinse quickly and pat them dry. You might want to lay them in front of a fan to remove excess moisture quickly.

drying herbs

You can dry herbs by hanging them in bunches, laying them on screens, or in shallow baskets. To dry herbs by hanging, tie the stalks into small bundles with string or twine. Hang them in a dry, well-ventilated place out of the sun. A shed or an attic is usually a good place. If you are drying herbs on screens or in baskets, remove the large leaves from their stems and spread them on the screens or baskets. Small leaves like thyme or savory, or needle-like ones like rosemary, should be left on their stems and laid on the screens.

To dry herbs for seed, be sure they are ripe. Herb seeds such as coriander, fennel or dill should be turning tan or light brown from green. Follow the same directions for hanging herbs to dry. Since they have a tendency to drop some of their seed as they dry, it is best to hang the bunches over a screen that will catch the seed. Or, you can hang each bundle in a paper bag with a few air holes cut in it, and the seeds will fall into the bag.

It may take from a few days to two weeks for the herbs to dry, depending on the climate and humidity. Check the herbs everyday; if they are left for too long, especially in humid weather, they will lose their green color and turn brown. When rubbed between your fingers, a dried herb should crackle and crumble. If it bends and is not crisp, there is still moisture in the leaf. To remove the last bit of excess moisture, preheat the oven to its lowest temperature, not over 200° F. Spread the herbs on baking sheets and place them in the warm oven for about five minutes. Repeat if necessary.

Alternatively, some herbs dry beautifully in the refrigerator. Italian or Sicilian oregano (*Origanum xmajoricum*), marjoram (*O. majorana*), thyme varieties, rosemary, dill and cilantro will dry green and fragrant. The sprigs must be completely free of water on the leaves and stems. Place small bunches in labeled, lunch-size paper bags. Fold the top of the bag down and lay it flat on an empty shelf. Turn the bag daily and gently shake the herbs so that air will circulate around leaf surfaces. The refrigerator's cool air keeps the volatile oils from evaporating. Drying time is variable. The process can take two to three weeks.

When the herbs are dried, carefully strip the whole leaves from their stems and pack them in clean jars, preferably dark glass, with tight-fitting lids. Do not crumble the leaves because this releases their essential oils. Pack them whole to retain the finest flavor. If the herbs are not completely dried when you pack them in jars they will mold and spoil. Label the jars and store them away from heat and light. Home-dried herbs can be stored in jars or tins about a year, when next season's crop will take their place.

freezing herbs

In our opinion, freezing most herbs does not yield good enough flavor for the effort. Freezing the leaves breaks down the cell structure so they often become mushy, and it tends to turn them dark. Tender-leaved herbs form ice crystals that make them watery after a month or two in the freezer. Sturdy-leaved herbs, such as sage and rosemary, have better flavor when dried. Some herbs are better preserved in vinegar. However, if you want to extend the season by a short time, or you have an abundance you just can't bear to throw away, we have found the following procedures are best for freezing.

Harvest and clean the herbs as instructed for drying. For the simplest method and the best flavor, freeze whole leaves. Remove the leaves from the stems and pack them in small, airtight freezer containers or pint freezer bags and label. If you want to pack the herbs in larger containers, first freeze the whole leaves individually on baking sheets, then transfer them to the containers. Remove the leaves as you need them; the bright green color will turn dark once they have been frozen.

Many herbs freeze well when chopped with a little oil. This method is good for preserving herb pastes for cooking (i.e.: pesto or *salsa verde*). We use olive oil for savory herbs. Small amounts of herbs like marjoram can be added to these blends when you plan to use them in cooked dishes. Or chop excess mints or lemon balm, mix them with a little vegetable oil—be sure to cover them with the oil—and you will have them when they are out-of-season to add to baked goods. Oil-frozen herbs are best stored in tightly-closed half-cup to cup-sized containers. *These herbs in oil must be kept in the freezer; do not keep them in the refrigerator because of the danger of botulism.*

herbs that we use most often
in our creative herbal home

The Herb of the Year, chosen by the International Herb Association (www.iherb.org) and supported by many other herbal organizations, is a tool for education and promotion of these important plants. Past and present Herbs of the Year are noted below. World origin of plants is noted for ethnobotanical interest.

Alkanet (*Alkanna tinctoria*) root is used as a natural red dye in our lip balm recipe. These plants originate from southern Europe and the Middle East. The herb is astringent, anti-bacterial and relieves itching. *Though alkanet root does have external uses, internal use is not advised because it contains pyrrolizidine alkaloids, which are toxic to the liver.*

Aloe vera (*Aloe vera*) plants hail from Africa, Arabia and the Cape Verde Islands along the Mediterranean coast. The gelatinous leaf juice is used topically to treat minor burns and wounds. The juice is antiseptic, digestive, insecticidal, larvicidal and emollient. The yellow juice, present just under the outer-leaf skin, is a powerful purgative when taken internally. *Persons suffering from spastic colon should not take aloe vera juice or other herbs containing anthraquinones as purgatives.*

Anise (*Pimpinella anisum*) is found in its wild state in central and southern Europe, Russia, northwest Africa and the Near East. It has a long history as a culinary and medicinal herb, valued for its leaves, seed and essential oil. We have used anise seed in bath blends for its fragrance and its reputation as an aphrodisiac. In cooking, it is used in desserts for its licorice-like flavor. Medicinally, anise improves digestion and is used as an expectorant.

Astragalus (*Astragalus membranaceus*) is a native of China. The dried root, called *huang qi* or *huang chi* ("yellow leader") is sold in long slices that are reminiscent of tongue depressors. These are decocted into tonic broths, soups and teas to boost the immune system, control night sweats, lower blood pressure and as a diuretic to treat edema. In Western medicine, studies have shown that astragalus helps boost production of white blood cells in cancer patients undergoing radiation and chemotherapy, resulting in improved recovery and longevity.

Basil (*Ocimum basilicum*) is a native of tropical Asia. It is a popular culinary herb with medicinal uses. It is included in our **herb potpourri sugar scrub** for its aroma. It is a nerve tonic that relieves stress, elevates the spirit and is good for oily skin and sore muscles. Basil was Herb of the Year for 2003.

Bay laurel (*Laurus nobilis*) trees and shrubs have fragrant evergreen leaves and are indigenous to southern Europe, the Canary Islands and the Azores. The fresh-dried leaves added to flour and grains are used to repel moths. Fresh or dried leaves are used both as a culinary seasoning and an antiseptic medicinal herb. Bay laurel was Herb of the Year for 2009.

Calendula (*Calendula officinalis*) is a cool season annual, native to Great Britain and southern Europe along the Mediterranean region. The flower petals are edible and used for their antiseptic, anti-inflammatory and anti-viral properties in the bath and in infusions, ointments and salves. The leaves have also been used to treat wounds. Internally, calendula has been used to treat liver problems, conjunctivitis, and delayed menses. Calendula was Herb of the Year for 2008.

German chamomile (*Matricaria recutita*) and **Roman chamomile** (*Chamaemelum nobile*) flowers are used in the bath and in tea for their calming, anti-inflammatory effects. Flower infusions are used as a rinse to bring out blond highlights in hair. Though these two plants are different species with different essential oils and chemistry, their flowers are used interchangeably. Chamazulene, an anti-inflammatory compound gives the essential oil of German chamomile a dark blue color when the flowers are steamed during the distillation process. German chamomile is native to western regions of Europe and the Azores. Roman chamomile is native to eastern regions of Europe, North Africa and western Asia.

Chickweed (*Stellaria media*) is a wild edible weed native to Europe. Though largely ignored by science and some popular herb writers, this terrific prolific plant is an anti-inflammatory herb. The stems, leaves and flowers have been used internally to ease the pain of rheumatism and externally to soothe itching and other skin discomforts. *Caution: Pregnant or nursing women should not eat large quantities of chickweed.*

Chile pepper (*Capsicum* spp.) is a seasoning and stimulating, antiseptic medicinal herb native to tropical America. Capsaicin, the primary active compound, causes local irritation to the skin, which increases blood flow to the area where it is applied. Taken internally, it is catabolic (warming), lowers cholesterol and may help us burn more calories.

Chives (*Allium schoenoprasum*) and (*A. tuberosum*) are culinary and medicinal herbs having similar health benefits as the other alliums, most especially garlic chives. Both have edible leaves and flowers and are used to flavor vinegars and food.

Chocolate, **cocoa** and **cocoa butter** (*Theobroma cacao*) come from the fermented, dried and roasted seeds of the plant. *Cacao is native to the tropical lowlands of Central and South America.* It contains over 300 chemical compounds, most noticeably the stimulating alkaloids theobromine and caffeine. Cocoa butter is solid at normal room temperature and melts at body temperature. This characteristic lends itself well to delicious lip balm formulations, though the balm will melt if you carry it in your pocket.

Citrus (*Citrus* spp.) peelings including grapefruit, lemon, lime and orange are used in home bath blends and as insect repellents. The essential oil of the rind is expressed and used for flavoring and fragrance. There are about 16 species of *Citrus* and they are native to southeastern Asia and the east Pacific islands. Recently, citrus oils have come under fire in the perfume and cosmetic industries because they contain **furocoumarins** (see **plant chemicals**) that cause phototoxicity (skin sensitivity, rashes and cell damage when exposed to UV rays). *Caution: Avoid sun and tanning beds when using these oils on the skin.*

Coltsfoot (*Tussilago farfara*) is a perennial, low-growing ground cover that is native to North Africa, western Asia and Europe. The leaves and flowers are astringent and contain mucilage that is useful for treating sores, insect stings, skin inflammation, eczema and dry skin. *Caution: This herb, especially the flowers, contains pyrrolizidine alkaloids that are poisonous to the liver. Internal use is not recommended.*

Comfrey (*Symphytum officinale* and *S.* x*uplandicum*) contains allantoin, a substance that speeds the healing of tissue and rosmarinic acid that is an anti-inflammatory. Wild comfrey grows in damp soil and is native to Europe and western Asia. It is an the creative herbal home

astringent herb we use in the bath, poultices and fomentations to heal bruises, broken bones and torn ligaments. *Caution: Comfrey is not recommended for internal use because of the presence of pyrrolizidine alkaloids, which can cause damage and cancerous tumors in the liver. Comfrey products should not be used on broken skin or be used by pregnant women, nursing mothers or children.*

Coriander (*Coriandrum sativum*), seed and leaf, is a culinary and medicinal herb native to southwest Asia and North Africa. The ground seed is used as a fomentation for treating hemorrhoids and sore joints. Whole seeds are added to herbal blends for fragrance.

Dandelion (*Taraxacum officinale*) is the familiar, yellow-flowering harbinger of spring that defies the efforts of those desiring perfect green lawns to poison it out of existence. Would our waterways be less polluted if we replaced the chemical-lawn services with wild crafters eager to harvest the beneficial leaves, flowers and roots of this determined plant? Dandelion thrives in all warm, temperate zones of the earth. The leaves and roots are astringent and bitter. Skin inflammations including acne, eczema and psoriasis are soothed with infusions of the leaves or decoctions of the roots. The leaves and roots are diuretic without depleting potassium levels in the body. Sipping a decoction of the roots may help to normalize blood sugar levels. The roots are best harvested and dried in the fall, when the bitter principle is low and the inulin level is highest. Inulin is useful as a prebiotic, providing high fiber and aiding the growth of beneficial flora in the intestines.

Dill (*Anethum graveolens*) is native to southern parts of Eurasia and is Herb of the Year for 2010. A culinary and medicinal herb, the seed and leaf are used as a diuretic and to treat hiccups, stomachache and colic.

14

Echinacea, or coneflower (*Echinacea* spp.), is a genus of useful and beautiful plants native to North America. The tops and roots are used in tea and tincture to boost the immune system, reduce the risk of sun damage to skin, fight viral infections and to heal minor wounds. The constituents include essential oils, glycosides, polysaccharides, inulin and caffeic acid esters. Echinacea was Herb of the Year in 2002. *Caution: Echinacea, when taken with other medications, including birth control drugs, may increase the risk of side effects. Persons with allergies to the Asteraceae family could suffer adverse effects when using this herb.*

Elderberry or **American Elder** (*Sambucus nigra* ssp. *canadensis*) is native to North America. The flowers, leaves and ripe, cooked fruit are used medicinally. The flowers and cooked fruit dry up mucus and soothe inflammation. The flowers are infused to make skin lotions. The leaves speed the healing of wounds and are a natural insecticide; they should only be used topically. Elderberry will be herb of the year 2012. *Caution: The leaves, seeds, bark, stems and root, as well as the unripe and raw fruit are toxic and should not be ingested. Only the berries, which must be cooked first and separated from the seed; and the blossoms are edible.*

Eucalyptus (*Eucalyptus globulus*) species are called gum trees in their native Australia. There are about 600 species of eucalyptus. Medicinally, the aromatic, astringent leaves of *E. globulus* are used to treat asthma, congestion and other breathing problems, as well as to lower fevers, treat fungal infections, nerve pain, sore throats, sprains, and bruises. Extracts are bactericidal, even controlling *staphylococci. Caution: Excessive use can cause headache or convulsions and can be fatal.*

Fennel (Foeniculum vulgare) leaves and seeds are culinary herbs, native to the Mediterranean areas of Europe. The aromatic seed, which contains the anise-scented essential oil, anethole, is used in bath blends for fragrance and to reduce inflammation. All parts of the plant smell like licorice and are used to flavor food and to treat digestive problems. Fennel was Herb of the Year for 1995.

Garlic (*Allium sativum* var. *sativum* and *A. sativum* var. ophioscorodon) cloves and leaves are used as a medicinal and culinary herb. Garlic has been cultivated for centuries all around the world but is native to central Asia. The cloves are antibiotic, anti-fungal, antiseptic and anti-viral. Garlic was Herb of the Year in 2004; we strongly believe (and practice) that garlic should be eaten everyday unless the individual has an allergy that would prevent its use.

Ginger (*Zingiber officinale*) springs from tropical Asia. The tubers are used fresh or dried for culinary and therapeutic purposes. Ginger is warming, antiseptic, analgesic and anti-spasmodic. It is a traditional remedy for digestive complaints, bronchitis, muscle spasm and rheumatism. *Caution: It should not be used by anyone suffering from digestive-tract ulcers, high fever or inflammatory skin conditions.*

Goldenseal (*Hydrastis canadensis*) is native to the eastern forest of the United States. It was listed as an endangered species in 1997 because native stands were over-harvested. The rhizomes have been used to dye fibers and are still used medicinally. The yellow color of its rhizomes is attributed to berberine, a strongly anti-bacterial and bitter alkaloid. *Caution: Pregnant or nursing women and persons with high blood pressure should not use goldenseal. The herb should not be used for more than two months because the strong anti-bacterial action kills beneficial intestinal flora.*

herbs

Jewelweed (*Impatiens capensis* and *I. pallida*) is a native annual
herb found growing along streams and springs in the eastern
United States. The juice from the entire plant is used to soothe
itchy skin conditions caused by poison ivy/oak, heat rash and
insect bites and stings. The active constituents of jewelweed
include lawsone and tannins. We crush the fresh plant and apply
the juice directly to skin irritations. We also preserve the juice in
apple cider vinegar to have it handy when needed. Jewelweed juice
may help prevent allergic reactions to toxic plant oils if applied
before exposure; however, the best prevention is avoiding direct
contact with toxic plants (and their smoke) and by washing shoes,
gloves, clothing, tools and pets with soap and cold water promptly
after plant contact has been made. Urushiol, the toxic oil of poison
ivy/oak, can spread from other surfaces to the skin.

Lavandin (*L.* x*intermedia*) is a group of hybrid lavenders, which
result from the cross between *L. angustifolia and L. latifolia*.
Lavandin plants are bred to resist fungal diseases of the genera
and to yield high quantities of essential oil for the fragrance
industry. The flowers, leaves and essential oils of lavandin are not
recommended for culinary use.

Lavender (*Lavandula angustifolia*) is native to India, mountain
ranges of the Mediterranean region and the Middle East.
Lavender contains linalool, linalyl acetate and perillyl alcohol.
It is antibiotic, anti-spasmodic on smooth muscle tissue and a
depressant to the central nervous system. We use the flowers and
leaves in bath blends for relaxation and fragrance. Both of us carry
a small vial of the essential oil of lavender with us everywhere we
go, to use as first aid for burns, wounds, headaches and nervous
tension. Lavender was Herb of the Year for 1999.

Lemon balm (*Melissa officinalis*) came originally from southern Europe, western Asia and North Africa. The leaf is used in tea, tincture and in the bath for its calming properties and pleasant lemon scent. Lemon balm is anti-bacterial, anti-spasmodic and anti-viral, and is used as an insect repellent and sedative. A double-blind study involving 115 patients with genital or oral herpes reported that lemon balm reduced the duration and incidence of outbreaks. It was Herb of the Year 2007, the year of this publication. *Caution: Pregnant or nursing women should consult a medical professional trained in the use of therapeutic herbs before taking lemon balm. Consult with your physician before taking lemon balm with other medications.*

Lemongrass (*Cymbopogon citratus* and *C. flexuosus*) is native to tropical southern India and Sri Lanka. *C. flexuosus*, East Indian lemongrass produces flowers and viable seed under cultivation in Arkansas and both varieties are easily grown as a tender perennial and propagated by division. Lemongrass is an insect repellent and culinary herb and is useful for a wide variety of therapeutic applications. The leaves can be infused in vinegar or water or tinctured in alcohol to create an insect repellent spray. Research has shown that lemongrass is anti-bacterial and anti-fungal. In the tropical places where it grows wild, folks use it in tea to treat fevers, depression, coughs and digestive complaints. Lemongrass has a long history of external use, usually as a poultice, for fighting fungal and bacterial skin infections.

Mint (*Mentha* spp.) leaves are used in tea and bath blends for their flavor, stimulating properties and fragrance. Menthol is the dominant essential oil in peppermint (*Mentha xpiperita*), while carvone is the dominant oil in spearmint (*M. spicata*). Therapeutic benefits include infusions of mint to aid digestion and reduce gas. Mint leaves are also taken in tea to treat headache, colds and fevers. Mint was Herb of the Year for 1998.

Monarda has about 15 or so relatives that are native to the forests of the eastern United States. **Horsemint** (*Monarda punctata*) is a good representative of the species because its leaves contain more antiseptic and anti-fungal thymol than thyme. Note that *M. fistulosa* is also called horsemint and contains less thymol. The red-flowered *M. didyma*, called Oswego tea and bee balm, has a high content of linalool and has much sweeter perfume and more agreeable flavor. Monarda was Herb of the Year for 1996.

Oregano (*Origanum* spp.) is a genus of about 20 species of plants native to Eurasia and North Africa. Common oregano (*O. vulgare*) grows rampantly in the garden and can be put to good use as an antiseptic herb. Besides being necessary for good Italian and Greek cuisine, the tea can be used to fight infections such as influenza because it contains the antiseptic essential oil, carvacrol. To research the possible uses for this herb, read James A. Duke's chapter on oregano in his book, *Herb-A-Day*. Origanum was Herb of the Year for 2005.

Patchouli (*Pogostemon cablin*) is native to India and Malaysia. We grow it as a houseplant, setting it on the patio or in the ground for the summer and then take it inside before temperatures get very cool at night in the fall. Though the essential oil is well known to baby boomers, the plant is rare in the U.S.. Those of us who grow it can study the ethno-botanical uses the plant has enjoyed for centuries. It has been used as an insect repellent for everything from bedbugs to leeches to moths. We use it in insect repellent preparations and find that applications are long lasting. Insects and mites do seem to avoid us when we are wearing it. The leaves have been poulticed on wounds and taken in tea for menstrual cramps, colds, headaches and digestive problems. In a clinical study in India, the essential oil was effective against many strains of bacteria and, most exciting, all fungi tested. It has been used to combat acne and impetigo.

American Pennyroyal (*Hedeoma pulegioides*) and **European pennyroyal** (*Mentha pulegium*) plants are used primarily as ornamentals and insect repellents in the garden in current times. Both contain the toxic compound, pulegone, which is poisonous to the liver and can be fatal when ingested in sufficient quantity. American pennyroyal is native to the dry woods of eastern North America. The tops of the plant and its essential oil have been used to induce sweating and aid digestion and as an expectorant. It also stimulates the uterus and has been used as an aid in childbirth and to induce the menses. European pennyroyal, which is also called pudding grass, is native to Europe and has culinary uses in a North England dish called black pudding, as well as a Spanish sausage seasoning. Its medicinal and insect-repellent uses are very similar to those of American pennyroyal.

Essential oil distilled from European pennyroyal (*M. pulegium*) is the one most often sold in the United States, though some products are marketed as "pennyroyal" without the plant species source listed on the label. American pennyroyal is rare and is not, to our knowledge, cultivated on farms, therefore, it is hard to imagine the possibility of finding *H. pulegioides* EO in the common market place. In the early 1990s, before Tina knew of the dangers of pulegone, she mail-ordered a large bottle of pennyroyal EO to make insect-repellent oils and vinegars. Though she has never experienced a negative reaction when using pennyroyal EO in these topical preparations, she is restricting the use of the pennyroyal left in her bottle to outdoor repellents to spray on the patio, yard and around doors and windows. She is careful not to get the oil on her skin or on that of her pets. We no longer purchase the essential oil of pennyroyal because it is potentially dangerous to our loved ones—we can repel pests with safer substances. *Caution: Both herbs can cause dermatitis when used externally and the essential oil can cause death when used internally. Pregnant or nursing women should not use either pennyroyal in any form; do not use it on your pets, even if the marketing information says that it is safe.*

Plantain (*Plantago major*) is a common volunteer in gardens, yards, in the woods and parks throughout the United States. A native of Europe and temperate Asia, plantain was called "white man's footsteps" because it became established as Europeans colonized other parts of the world. Most plantain species enjoy a host of folk uses wherever they grow. Plantain is a good substitute for comfrey in healing salves. It is anti-microbial and astringent and makes a soothing wash for poison ivy/oak rash. One clinical study revealed that the seed and/or leaves of plantain, when taken with water one-half hour before meals, reduces bad cholesterol, increases good cholesterol and restricts the absorption of lipids (fats) in the intestines.

Red clover (*Trifolium pratense*) is native to the eastern sections of the Mediterranean and Asia. An infusion of the flowers is traditionally used as a diuretic; a tonic "blood purifier"; as a wash for sore eyes, eczema and psoriasis; and taken in tea for coughs. Red clover contains isoflavones (plant estrogens) that attach to estrogen receptors in the body. Studies indicate that red clover extract increases the elasticity of arteries and so may improve cardiovascular health. This simple, beautiful and harmless herb could offer nutritional support in the fight against cancer.

Rose (*Rosa* spp.) is a genus of plants containing about 150 species
that are native to northern temperate climates throughout the
world. As an astringent, rose petals tighten the skin and dry up
weeping wounds and rashes. We grow fragrant varieties and use
them in the bath and for facial treatments. Rose hips, the fruits that
are born from the flowers, are high in vitamin C.

Rosemary (*Rosmarinus officinalis*) is native to mountainous
coastal regions all around the Mediterranean Sea. The leaves and
flowers contain essential oils, especially rosmarinic acid, that are
analgesic, anti-inflammatory, anti-microbial and antioxidant. We
use the essential oil in aromatherapy products and the bath, as well
as using the herb in the tub, for its stimulating, memory-enhancing
effects. Rosemary was Herb of the Year for 2000.

Sage (*Salvia officinalis*) is a hardy, woody sub-shrub native to
the Mediterranean region and North Africa. *Salvia* is a genus
with representative species all over the world. Many of them
are revered, sacred plants and are called by the common name,
sage. Garden sage contains the powerful compound, thujone that
controls profuse perspiration and dries up lactation. Sage tea is a
traditional remedy for sore gums and throat, skin infections and
insect stings and for sharpening the memory. Currently, *Salvia*
species are being researched for their antioxidant properties,
specifically for the prevention or treatment of Alzheimer's disease.
Sage was Herb of the Year for 2001. *Caution: Pregnant or nursing
women should not take sage internally. It should not be taken
internally in large amounts or for extended periods because of the
potentially toxic side-effects of thujone.*

Scented geranium (*Pelargonium* spp.) is a genus containing
about 230 species of tender perennials native to South Africa. In
the horticultural trade, they have been given names that suggest

individual aromas and possibilities for use. For example, the leaves and flowers of 'Prince of Orange', 'Lemon Crispum', 'Nutmeg' and rose geranium are useful in the bath, in cooking and around the home to impart fragrance. The only scented geranium EO sold is rose, which we use in many homemade products. Scented geraniums must not be confused with the familiar *Geranium* genus; though related, their uses are distinctly different. Scented Geranium was Herb of the Year for 2006.

St.-John's-wort (*Hypericum* spp.) is a genus of annual, perennial, shrubs and trees native to western Asia, Europe and North America. Common St.-John's-wort (*H. perforatum*), a native of Europe that has escaped cultivation in the U.S., is the infamous antidepressant herb brought to our attention by the media in June 1997. There are seven native American species of Hypericum growing in the Arkansas Ozarks. The leaves and flowers are harvested when the plants are in bloom. Hypericin's antidepressive, tissue-healing and anti-viral actions are attributed to varying levels of the glycosides hypericin, hyperforin, adhyperforins and proanthocyadinins. The freshly dried flowers are infused in oil to make healing ointments and salves for burns and abrasions. *Caution: Ingestion may cause phototoxicity in sensitive individuals.*

Tansy (*Tanacetum vulgare*) is a native of Europe. The leaves smell and taste acrid and bitter. Tansy leaves and flowering tops, harvested as the seed begins to ripen, contain varying amounts of pyrethrins. Pyrethrins are toxic to the nervous system of insects. It repels or knocks them down without apparent harm to mammals and vertebrates. The herb is especially valuable to repel ants and flies. *Caution: Tansy contains variable levels of the toxic compound, thujone. It must be handled with gloves and a high measure of respect. Ingestion can produce convulsions and* *psychotic behavior. Though tansy is listed on the FDA's GRAS (generally recognized as safe) list, it carries the restriction that it can only be used as a flavoring if it is free of thujone. It is illegal to sell the herb as food or medicine. The EO is not safe. Ingesting one-half ounce of the essential oil can be fatal within a few hours.*

Tea (*Camellia sinensis*) is a native of Southeast Asia. Green tea leaves are steamed and dried. Oolong tea leaves have been slightly fermented before they are dried. The leaves are fully fermented and roasted to make black tea. Tea is being touted for its antioxidant properties. We use astringent green or black tea to tighten skin, temporarily reducing the appearance of wrinkles and in foot soak blends for the tannic acid they contain.

Thyme (*Thymus vulgaris*) is just one of some 350 species in the genus. Thymes are native to dry grasslands, soil rich in lime throughout Europe and Asia. Common thyme is native to the eastern regions bordering the Mediterranean Sea. An infusion of thyme is traditionally used to quiet coughs, settle stomach and other digestive complaints and to relieve menstrual problems. The bacterium *Helicobacter pylori*, is linked to stomach ulcers and is killed by extracts of thyme under laboratory conditions. Garden thyme, along with other herbs including American dittany (*Cunila origanoides)* and horsemint (*Monarda punctata*), contain the compound, thymol, in their essential oils. Thyme was Herb of the Year for 1997. *Caution: Thymol is potentially toxic and is a uterine stimulant. Pregnant and nursing women should restrict their use of thyme to the culinary.*

White oak (*Quercus alba*) trees are native to the eastern United States. The inner bark, leaves and acorns contain tannic acid. It hardens the proteins in the skin and is antiseptic, anti-fungal and anti-bacterial.

Wormwood (*Artemesia absinthium*) hails from Europe and temperate Asia. Absinthium means "without sweetness." Extracts of the plant contain sesquiterpene lactones and the anti-inflammatory pigment, azulene. The leaf is very bitter and its essential oil contains thujone, a neurotoxin. Southernwood (*A. abrotanum*) has similar constituents and uses to wormwood. We use these *Artemesia* species as insect repellents to keep moths out of our drawers and in bundles attached to the screen door to discourage bugs from following us into the house. The leaves provide a quick garden poultice for insect stings. Traditionally, infusions of the herb are used to stimulate the uterus in cases of slow or painful menses and as a vermifuge to expel intestinal worms. The tea, if taken, should only be used on a short-term basis in very small amounts. *Caution: Pregnant and nursing women or children should not ingest wormwood.*

Yarrow (*Achillea millefolium*) is native to northern temperate climates. The astringent and antiseptic leaves and flowers have long been used to staunch the bleeding of wounds and, internally, to treat fevers. The essential oil contains the anti-inflammatory compound azulene.

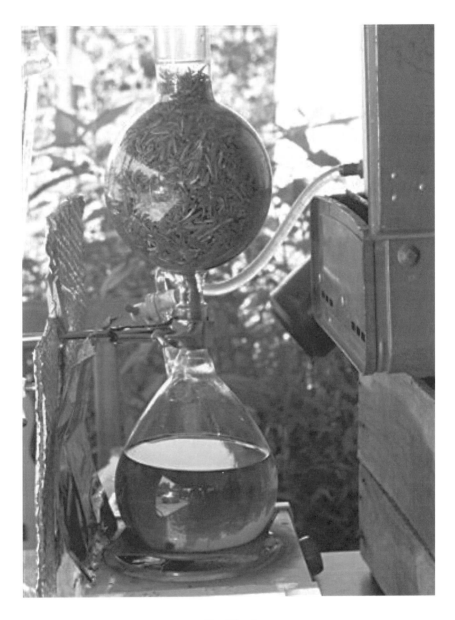

rosemary distillation process

plant chemicals

Having some understanding of the chemicals in plants is useful to those creating an herbal home. It is a matter of personal responsibility to know and understand as much as possible about the chemical properties of plants and their essential oils. The freedom to purchase, use, and make herbal products comes with personal responsibility. We all must practice safe procedures and make informed decisions about the natural substances that we introduce into our immediate environment, especially in and on our bodies. Some regulators would take this responsibility away and restrict our use of therapeutic herbs to those prescribed by a physician. While plants are potent and chemically complex, they belong to the earth, as do we. To regulate what we consume for therapeutic purposes is an attack on our civil liberties. Let us endeavor to learn all that we can about the world of herbs and keep our freedom to obtain the herbs and essential oils that we choose to use on the open market.

Laypersons, even seasoned herbalists, don't always know the definition of words used in the language of chemistry and may miss important clues or safety issues. This chapter, arranged alphabetically, attempts to explain some of the words we come across as we study our herbals. Don't worry if you cannot imagine combining elemental atoms. Read through this to see if you can relate what you know about plants through your senses with the descriptions of the chemistry.

Chemical compounds are combinations of elemental atoms such as carbon, oxygen, hydrogen and nitrogen. These atoms and their compounds have properties, that is, they do things that can be predicted. Chemists study plants at a microscopic level. They identify the elemental atoms, molecules and compounds and isolate them from one another. As the isolates are discovered, they are named so that people have a common language to talk about, study, test and use them.

Acids are created when hydrogen combines with other elements such as carbon or oxygen and the hydrogen atom casts off ions. The more hydrogen ions that come loose and are present in the compound, the stronger the acid is. When hydrogen is attached to a single carbon atom, hydrogen ions do not break away very much. When hydrogen is attached to oxygen, it is called a *hydroxyl* and there is only a small chance of ions breaking loose. The acid content of ethyl alcohol is barely perceptible by chemists. However, when hydroxyl attaches to a benzene ring (six carbon atoms linked together in a ring with three double bonds), as they do in many plant constituents, the acids are stronger but still mild compared to many chemicals such as muriatic acid. Acids are present in plant parts as either mineral salts or as esters. Acid names usually end in "ic."

Sorrel (*Oxalis acetosella*) is a good example of an herb that contains mineral salts. When we taste sorrel, we can taste the sour acid. "Salt of sorrel" is an old chemistry term for the chemical compound, acid potassium oxalate, which is used as a solvent for ink. This compound was called "salt of sorrel" because the same chemistry is found in sorrel. Sorrel contains a polybasic acid whose make-up is described below. Early chemists used the term "essential salt" to describe the powder obtained when they crystallized plant juices.

Plant acids are categorized according to how many hydroxyl groups are in the molecule. Simple straight-chain acids with one hydroxyl group are called monobasic acids. Valeric acid from valerian and formic acid from stinging nettles are examples of monobasic acids.

Straight-chained molecules with more than twelve carbon atoms make up the nutritionally important poly-unsaturated and saturated fats. In chemistry, these are called "fixed oils". Fixed oils are not easily volatilized and are comprised of glycerol and three fatty acids. These acids are in seed oils such as almond, olive and sunflower seed that we use to make herbal oils.

There are many polybasic acids. These are made up of chains of more than one hydroxyl group. Oxalic acid in sorrel and tannic acid in tea are polybasic acids. It is interesting that the acid in sorrel tastes sour and the acid in tea tastes a little bitter or astringent.

Aromatic acids are a large and medically important group. Benzoic acid is a simple aromatic acid that has a benzene ring and a hydroxyl group. Gum benzoic and balsam of Peru are two examples of herbs with aromatic acids. Phenol is often referred to as carbolic acid and was first isolated in coal tar.

Prussic or hydrocyanic acid is completely different than any other acid. The toxin is present in the seed and other plant parts of many useful plants. Beneath the epidermis, in the mesaphyll cells, there are enzymes that combine with the hydrocyanic acid molecules when the plant parts are damaged. Fruits with pits, such as peach, cherry, apricot and elderberry contain hydrocyanic acid. *Caution is required when making jams, jellies and shrub with these fruits. It is very important to strain out the pits and discard them safely.* Some kinds of lima beans, flax, spinach, sorghum, and a host of other plants contain hydrocyanic acid but we have found no reports of human fatalities caused by eating these foods. However, there is a report that a person died from eating 1/2 cup apple seeds.

When ruminants, such as cows, sheep, goats and llamas graze on certain grasses, various weeds, elderberry and chokecherry which contain hydrocyanic acid, they fall victim to cyanide poisoning.

Since they have multiple stomachs and chew cud, there is ample time and rumen bacteria to breakdown and release cyanide from the plant material into the bloodstream. Affected animals salivate, stagger, have trouble breathing, convulse and die very quickly. Animals with only one stomach, such as humans, are not as apt to be killed by eating plants that contain hydrocyanic acid. Digestive acids usually neutralize the toxin before it can do fatal harm.

Albumin is a class of protein substances present in animal tissues such as blood, milk and got its name from egg whites. Albumin is in most plant tissues but plays an especially important role in seeds. It feeds and cushions the little embryo inside the seed coat. Bark and roots contain a whole lot of this protein.

We need to know that albumin coagulates when subjected to heat, alcohol and strong acids. It dissolves in cold water. If you want to prepare a decoction using bark, roots or seed, chop or crush the herb and soak it in cold water to soften the tissues and dissolve the albumin. Then slowly bring the water to a boil. If roots or seeds are put into boiling water at the beginning of the process, the albumin will coagulate all at once and interfere with the extraction of desired plant constituents.

Alcohol, chemically speaking, is a molecule that contains one or more hydroxyl group (one hydrogen atom and one oxygen atom), which attaches itself to carbon atoms. Diluted ethyl alcohol, such as vodka, is the solution we use to make tinctures. Alcohol names usually end in "ol".

The alcohols in essential oils are divided into **monoterpenols**, **sesquiterpenols** and **diterpenols**. When a hydroxyl molecule attaches to a terpene, the result is a **monoterpenol**. Menthol from peppermint and linalool from lavender and basil are monoterpenols.

They are non-irritating yet strongly anti-bacterial, anti-viral and stimulating. When a hydroxyl group attaches to a **sesquiterpene**, the result is a **sesquiterpenol**. These are non-irritating and are used as tonics. Farnesol is an alcohol found in many essential oils including citronella and lemongrass and contributes to the insecticidal properties of these oils. To follow the pattern, **diterpenols** are formed when a hydroxyl group attaches to a diterpene. These molecules, having so many carbon atoms, are very heavy and are rarely found in essential oils because they are not carried up into the distillation by the steam. However, they are important because they resemble human hormones and have a balancing effect on the endocrine system.

Aldehydes are present in some essential oils and are formed by oxidation of alcohols. Note that their names end in "al." They are often lemon-scented. Citral from lemon balm and citronellal from lemongrass, lemon eucalyptus and lemon balm are examples of the very aromatic aldehydes. They can irritate the skin but are calming, tonic and anti-fungal. Aldehydes are not soluble in water but are soluble in ethyl alcohol.

Alkaloids from plants are molecules made up of carbon, hydrogen and nitrogen that can combine with organic acids to form soluble salts. They are soluble in water and somewhat soluble in alcohol. Some plant alkaloids are extremely poisonous and/or have strong psychological and physiological effect on the mind and body. Alkaloid names usually end in 'ine'. Examples of familiar alkaloids are morphine (from poppies), nicotine (from tobacco) and theobromine (from chocolate). Comfrey contains pyrrolizidine alkaloids that are toxic to the liver. Calendula petals contain the alkaloid calenduline.

Anthraquinones are plant constituents that act as purgatives in the digestive system. They are usually combined with sugar molecules in the plant and are called glycosides. Anthraquinones are present in aloe vera latex, senna and cascara sagrada and are marketed as natural laxatives and "dieter's tea." When you see this word listed as a specific plant constituent, be aware that you are messing with some powerful purgatives. As these substances move through the digestive tract, they stimulate contractions in the intestinal walls. Gripping pains in the lower abdomen are common. Carminative herbs such as peppermint are administered with purgatives to ease this side effect. *Caution: Persons with constipation due to spastic colon should not take herbs that contain anthraquinones. All persons should leave the use of anthraquinones as a last resort in the treatment of constipation. They are very strong acting, unpleasant and may cause dependency with long-term use.*

Bitter compounds are important because the characteristic flavor stimulates the digestive system and other glandular activity in the body. Bitters are taken to help the stomach secrete digestive fluid to increase the digestion of food and to stimulate the appetite. Bitter compounds are soluble in water and alcohol. Calendula petals, gentian and hops are examples of gentle bitter herbs. Wormwood and tansy are examples of bitter herbs that contain toxic compounds and should not be taken internally without strict supervision of a qualified medical or herbal practitioner.

Coloring matter is the pigmentation in plants. At the top of the list is chlorophyll, which makes photosynthesis possible. Chlorophyll helps cleanse and detoxify cells in the body. Olive oil contains chlorophyll and is an excellent solvent for medicinal herbs. **Polyphenols** are responsible for the coloring in some plants.

Carotenoid pigments are an important class of compounds found in calendula, cayenne, chickweed and a whole host of other herbs, fruits and vegetables. Some carotenoids are converted to vitamin A (beta-carotene) in the body and some are antioxidants. Antioxidants are substances that neutralize the harmful effects of free radicals in the body. Free radicals are groups of atoms with the element oxygen attached that are introduced into the body through pollutants. They do cell damage, harm the immune system and can cause infection and cancer. The bottom line is, use nature's palette (eat all colors of fruits and vegetables) to please your palate and protect your person.

Coumarins in plants have the aroma of new mown hay with a hint of vanilla. Sweet woodruff, lavender, meadow sweet and white clover contain coumarins. Synthetic coumarins are the basis of the anti-coagulant drug and rodent poison, warfarin. Coumarins thin the blood by interfering with vitamin K metabolism, and so are used therapeutically as anti-clotting agents. Many coumarins act as vasodilators by relaxing the smooth muscles in blood vessels, allowing them to dilate. Coumarins are also anti-bacterial and anti-spasmodic. When warnings are given about using plants that contain coumarins, often it is the furocoumarins, (also called furanocoumarins) to which they are referring. Please read the entry about these compounds below.

Caution: Patients who are taking warfarin drugs must consult with their doctors if they take herbs such as ginseng, ginger, garlic and ginkgo. These herbs and foods may increase blood pressure and therefore increase the risk of bleeding or hemorrhage. Pregnant women and heart patients must be very cautious and aware of the herbs that affect the circulatory system.

Enzymes are present in live animal and plant cells. They are chemical catalysts that break down or build up the molecules of specific substances or groups. They are soluble in water and insoluble and rendered inactive in alcohol. Enzymes are destroyed by moist heat. When making medicine we are often concerned with preserving glycosides, the "active ingredients" in the preparation. Alcohol or boiling water stops the destructive activity of enzymes on glycosides.

Essential oils are contained in sacs in plants. These substances are chemically complex and are not really "oils" as we might think of the word in relation to what we use in our kitchens or automobiles. They are lighter than water, and so float to the top of the surface. They do not leave a grease spot and they evaporate, or volatilize into the atmosphere quickly. They are made up of straight chain hydrocarbons, terpenoids and/or benzene derivatives. Scientists isolate compounds from essential oils and these compounds have many names and have been studied for their activity. The following are just a few of the common essential oil compounds, with definitions, that we find referred to in our herbal texts.

Anethole is present in the essential oil of fennel, star anise and anise seed. It appears as shining, white crystalline scales when the essential oils are cooled. The crystals smell strongly of anise seed and are used in carminative and expectorant medications.

Camphors are components extracted from essential oils that are somewhat solid or crystallized but are easily melted. They are separated from distilled essential oils and sold separately for use in medicinal and therapeutic agents, household products and industry. The essential oils are first put through a cooling process and

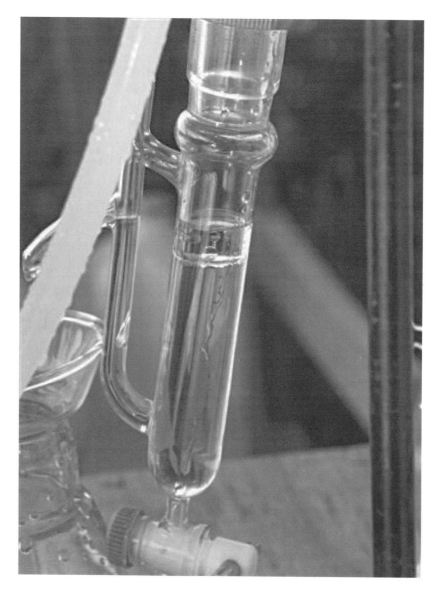

in the distillation process, the distillate is in the bottom of the tube and the essential oil floats on top

then crystals of the camphor are added to the oil to speed up the crystallization process. Camphor is extracted from the wood of the camphor tree (*Cinnamomum camphora*). Camphors are insoluble in water and soluble in alcohol.

Carvacrol is an antiseptic phenol and a constituent of many essential oils, particularly oregano, savory, and wild bergamot (*Monarda fistulosa*).

Carvone is the main constituent of spearmint and is a ketone. It is used for children's maladies and for flavoring in foods and dental products.

D-Limonene is isolated from the essential oil of citrus fruits. It is an insect repellent. *Caution: It must not be used on the skin in the presence of UV rays and should never be used on dogs and cats.*

Linalool is an alcohol and is present in the essential oils of basil and lavender, among other herbs. It is absorbed through the skin and mucous membranes. Once in the circulatory system, this substance depresses the nervous system, reduces agitation and sensation of pain.

Menthol is a monoterpenoid alcohol extracted from peppermint oil. It is active against viral organisms including herpes and West Nile virus and is strongly anti-bacterial. Menthol is a refrigerant that reduces the sensation of pain and itching. It is used in muscle liniments and upset- stomach remedies. Everyone recognizes menthol as a flavoring in toothpaste, candy and gum.

Rosmarinic acid is a compound isolated from the essential oils of many herbs in the mint family including rosemary and sage. It stops perspiration and is active against viral and bacterial organisms.

Thujone smells of camphor, and when over-used, it is a neurotoxin that is addictive and produces hallucinations. Garden sage, tansy and wormwood contain thujone in their essential oils. Thujone is a ketone.

Thymol is present in the essential oils of garden thyme, West African basil (*Ocimum gratissimum*) and horsemint among others. It often occurs in plants that contain carvacrol. To extract the thymol, essential oils are infused with a warm, alkaline solution of sodium hydroxide (lye). Terpenes and other matter that do not dissolve, float to the top and are removed. Then the alkaline thymol solution is treated with hydrochloric (muriatic) acid that produces the final product, crystalline phenol. This powerfully antiseptic **phenol** is antibiotic, anti-fungal, anti-inflammatory, antitussive (relieves coughs) and antioxidant. *Caution: When thymol is isolated from essential oils or is produced in its pure form, it is toxic. Essential oils that contain thymol produce a warming or burning sensation to the skin when applied neat and should be well diluted in carrier oils before using. Thyme oil is downright uncomfortable and burning when it is applied to broken skin or mucous membranes.*

Esters are formed when molecules of acid and alcohol combine in the laboratory or in biological life. Both contain the elements hydrogen and oxygen. When they merge, water, H_2O is created and eliminated from the tissue. The properties of both of the original molecules are cancelled out. What remains are colorless, volatile liquids with mostly pleasant aromas and flavors. Esters are responsible for the fragrance in flowers, fruits and essential oils. Their names end in "yl" (pronounced "eel") followed by ester group name. Important esters include linalyl acetate from lavender and bergamot. Methyl salicylate, a toxic ester, is found in birch and wintergreen.

Flavonoids are a group of polyphenolic molecules that are present in all plant pigments except green and are contained in all flowering plants. They are strongly antioxidant. Contained within this group, named according to their chemical structure, are flavanols, flavanones, isoflavones, catechins, anthocyanidins and chalcones. Many flavonoids are present in flower pigments. Others are attached to sugars in other plant parts. Almost all flavonoids assist vitamin C with its antioxidant functions. Soybeans, dark chocolate and herbs such as red clover flowers contain these compounds, possibly as a natural defense against insect pests.

Flavones are notable flavonoids because they are phenolic compounds found in the leaves of about 50% of flowering plants. Flavone comes from the Latin word "flavus" which means yellow. Bioflavonoids always accompany vitamin C in nature. Flavonoids stimulate the heart and circulatory system, are diuretic, and anti-spasmodic. Calendula petals contain flavonoids that help new capillaries grow on damaged skin tissue

Furocoumarins, also called furanocoumarins, are present in the oils of celery, parsley, angelica and other members of the Apiaceae family of plants, as well as citrus peels, fig sap, rue and some composite family plants. The skin is exposed to the oils of these plants through application of homemade insect repellents or fragrances; by squeezing limes, oranges or lemons for their juice; applying tanning lotions and creams; harvesting, pruning, using a "weed whacker" or "string trimmer" on plants that contain furocoumarins.

When the skin is simultaneously exposed to sunlight or tanning lights, (UVA radiation) an allergic reaction occurs that is called phototoxicity. The furocoumarins absorb the energy of photons and releases it into skin cells, causing damage to the DNA. The first reaction comes on quickly, between 15 minutes to two hours. The skin begins to burn and itch. Washing with cold water eases the sensation but does not stop the discomfort completely.

Sweating in the hot sun exacerbates the reaction. After 24 hours, a rash may develop with blistering and strange, red markings on the skin. In one to two weeks, skin pigment changes (called hyperpigmentation) can develop, especially in fair-skinned people and last for months or years. In addition, affected areas may remain sensitive to sun exposure for several gardening seasons. Gardening and farming exposure risks are highest during the mid-to-late summer when plant oils are strongest.

Caution: To protect the skin against the damage, wear long sleeves and trousers, gloves and a hat. Know the plants that contain furocoumarins in your garden and take precautions to keep the oils off of skin exposed to sun. Do not wear products containing citrus out-of-doors or under tanning lights.

Glycosides are active principles in plant drugs. The names of almost all glycosides end in "in". For example, echinacin B and inulin are glycosides in *Echinacea purpurea*.

Glycoside compounds are made up of a sugar part attached to a non-sugar part called an aglycone. When the sugar part is glucose, the compounds are called glucosides; they have a neutral pH. Glycosides become active when they react with water and are metabolized by enzymes present in neighboring cells. It is important to preserve fresh plant material in alcohol or properly dry it to stop the destruction of glycosides by enzymes. There are varying degrees of solubility in glycosides. Nearly all are soluble in alcohol and this is why many herbalists believe that echinacea tincture is more effective than echinacea tea.

Glycosides are divided into categories according to their actions on the body. Cardiac glycosides are so named because these affect the contractions of the heart. Foxglove (*Digitalis purpurea*) contains the cardiac glycosides digitoxin, digoxin and gitoxin.

Cyanogenic glycosides are potentially poisonous plant principles that affect the heart rate, are sedative and effect respiration. The uncooked fruits of elderberry and the pits of cherries, peaches and plums are examples of plants that contain cyanogenic glycosides.

Mustard is in a separate glycoside category, distingished because the sugar molecule is attached to a sulfur atom instead of an oxygen atom. We are familiar with the effect that those sulfur atoms bring to food—from the slightly sharp flavor of ground mustard seeds to the penetrating, burning vapor released into the sinuses and eyes while eating Chinese mustard. Mustard plasters have been used as expectorants.

Saponin glycosides foam when shaken with water. "Bouncing Bet" (*Saponaria officinalis*) is a good example of a plant that contains saponin glycosides.

Gums are carbohydrates that exude from some plants. They are water-soluble. When dissolved in water they form emollient, soothing ointment or a demulcent substance that soothes mucous membranes.

They may have mucilage or can be readily softened to form an adhesive paste. Gums are not soluble in alcohol. Examples are acacia, aloe vera and tragacanth.

Gum-resins exude from plants, especially trees and shrubs and are either gums that are soluble in water or resins that are soluble in alcohol. Examples are myrrh and asafoetida. Gum-resins are sticky acrid, aromatic, astringent and antiseptic.

Isoflavones, from soybeans, red clover and most beans that we eat are phytoestrogens. The active compounds are similar enough to human estrogen "but weaker" that researchers speculate that the isoflavones attach to estrogen receptors in the body. This results in less estrogen in the system, that can contribute to PMS and post-menopausal discomfort. Isoflavones have a compound that is similar to the human hormone estrogen that fits into the estrogen receptors found around the body. This modality in the body is also thought to help reduce the risk of breast cancer. There is controversy about the health benefits of isoflavones in soy products. We'll eat some tofu every now and then and let the scientists work out the details.

Ketones are created when a single oxygen atom attaches to a carbon atom to form a unit and then, that all-new unit hooks up with a hydrocarbon compound. Sounds explosive doesn't it? Well, some ketones are highly flammable and can be toxic to the nervous system. Whether they be friend or foe, ketone names end in "one." For example, the toxic ketones are thujone, which is in tansy, sage and wormwood, and pulegone that is in pennyroyal. Gentler acting ketones include carvone in spearmint oil and menthone in peppermint.

Mucilages are carbohydrates. They are soluble in water and insoluble in alcohol. It is important to know if plant material contains mucilage and use only as much alcohol as needed to preserve the extract. Comfrey is a plant with mucilage that makes a goopy alcohol tincture. Calendula contains mucilage.

Oils (commonly referred to as fixed oils by botanists and scientists) have a characteristic greasy feel and are distinctly different chemically than essential oils. They are composed of the three elementary fats: olein, stearin and palmitin. Each of these is made up of fatty acids and glycerin. Fixed oils (as opposed to volatile oils) are soluble in chloroform, ether, and in volatile oils or other fats. When fixed oils are present in plant material, solvency of alcohol and water preparations are compromised. Echinacea and flax seed contains fatty acids.

Olive oil called "sweet oil" in old herbals, is used as an herbal oil to great advantage. It is high in chlorophyll, fatty acids and vitamin E. Expeller or cold-pressed extra-virgin olive oil is the healthy and tasty choice for food and medicine.

Wheat germ oil is rich in vitamins B, E and protein. It is used in ointments to extend the shelf life of these preparations because of its antioxidant qualities. Wheat germ oil is added in a 10% solution after the ointment has cooled. Shelf life of herbal oils and ointments can be extended from only two weeks without the wheat germ oil to about six months with the wheat germ oil.

Phenol is also a word most often used for carbolic acid, an antiseptic substance isolated from coal tar and introduced as a surgical antiseptic by Sir Joseph Lister. Chemically it is made of carbon, hydrogen and oxygen atoms and expressed as C_6H_5OH. When a hydroxyl unit attaches to a ring of carbon atoms, it is a phenol, regardless of the source from whence the atoms came. Thymol and carvacrol are two examples of phenols extracted from the essential oils of plants. *Caution: Do not use herbs and essential oils with phenols on cats. Oregano oil is an example. They cannot digest these substances and ingestion can cause illness and death.*

Polyphenols are chemical substances that can be isolated from plants. The prefix, poly, indicates that there is more than one phenol group in each molecule. It is a hydroxyl group (OH) bonded to a phenyl ring and they are aromatic compounds.

Polyphenols are divided into the categories of tannins and phenylpropanoids (lignins and flavonoids). White oak bark contains tannic acid, which is a polyphenol.

Saponins, like soap, foam when the plant part is crushed and mixed with water. Saponins are glycosides. They hold fats and resins in suspension in aqueous solutions of water and diluted alcohol. Some saponins, such as those found in wild yam and fenugreek, appear to serve as precursors to female sex hormones.

Still other saponins have been categorized as triterpenoid saponins. Triterpenoids are a class of hydrocarbons produced by plants with six isoprene units and three carbon rings. The compounds are not well studied and are very complex. These are found in many plants including astragalus, calendula petals, chickweed and soybeans. Tri-terpenoid saponins are important lung and adrenal gland remedies.

There are also toxic saponins called sapotoxins. Plants containing this toxin include "Bouncing Bet" *(Saponaria officinalis)* and agave *(Agave lecheguil')* both of which are toxic to sheep, goats and cattle.

Starches are common in plant tissues and are not soluble in common solvents. They are responsible for some of the cloudiness in teas and tinctures. Starch particles swell in boiling water and, in large enough quantity, form a mucilaginous paste. Examples are cornstarch, arrowroot and tapioca.

Sugars are called saccharides from the Greek word *sakcharon*. They can be simple units called monosaccharides, taste sweet, and be soluble in water and dilute alcohol. Two to ten sugar units linked together are called oligosaccharides. When very many sugar units are linked together, they are called polysaccharides.

Polysaccharides do not taste sweet and are not very soluble. They are in cellulose, the support system of cells, are in starches that make up food reservoirs, and are in gums that ooze out to protect plants when they are wounded. The polysaccharides in echinacea root extracts are antibiotic. Echinacea also contains glucose, sucrose and fructose. Calendula contains polysaccharides.

Tannins are in the bark and leaves of many kinds of plants. They have an astringent taste. Protein is coagulated when it is exposed to tannins. The skin surface feels smooth and mucous membranes stop or slow secretions. Echinacea, green tea and white oak bark are examples of herbs that contain tannins. Because tannins are so common in plants, they are of particular interest to people making tinctures. Tannins are very soluble in water and soluble in alcohol and glycerin. Precipitates are formed when tannins combine with the nitrogen in alkaloids and minerals. Dark solids will settle to the bottom of the container. *This sediment can contain alkaloids in a dangerous concentration level. This is why it is necessary to shake a tincture twice daily during maceration. It is also important to shake the finished tincture before taking the medicine.* Vegetable glycerin can be added to the menstruum to bind the tannins, preventing them from precipitating any alkaloids.

Terpenes, monoterpenes, sesquiterpenes and **diterpenes** are classifications of isoprene units found in essential oils. Terpene is an all-inclusive word for all of the isoprene units that make up an essential oil. Isoprene units are molecules made up of five carbon atoms and 8 hydrogen atoms with the molecular formula C_5H_8. These units build up chains and are classified sequentially by size. A **monoterpene** has two isoprene units joined together with the molecular formula $C_{10}H_{16}$. These can irritate the skin but are important because they can kill some germs. Geraniol and limonene are examples of monoterpenes.

Sesquiterpenes are made up of three isoprene units with the molecular formula $C_{15}H_{24}$ and are important because they stimulate glands in the liver and are anti-bacterial, anti-spasmodic and anti-inflammatory. Wormwood contains sesquiterpenes. The prefix "sesqui" means one-and-one-half. **Diterpenes** are made up of four isoprene units with the molecular formula $C_{20}H_{32}$. They are heavy molecules and so don't make it into essential oil distillations very often. They are expectorant, purgative and may have anti-fungal and anti-bacterial properties. The prefix "di" means twice.

Waxes are compounds comprised of alcohol and fatty acids (but differ from fats because they contain no glycerin). These compounds are on plant surfaces and repel water. Waxes are brittle when cold and melt when they are heated. You can see wax floating on the surface of herbal infusions as the water cools. Beeswax is used to make ointments and plasters. Carnauba wax is extracted from the salt palm.

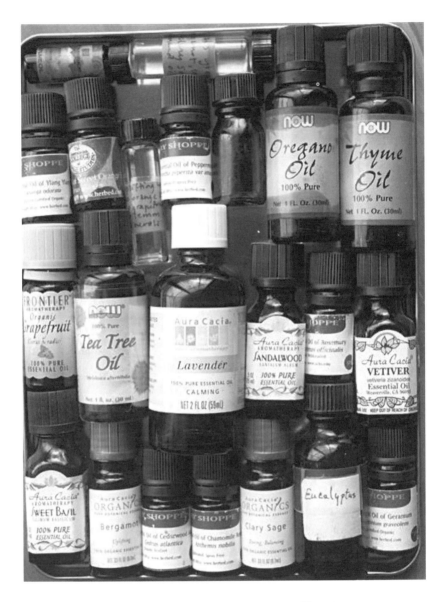

some essential oils in our collection

essential oils

Essential oils (which we refer to as EOs, as do many in the trade) are highly concentrated "essences" of single plant species, extracted by distillation or, in the case of citrus oils, by expression. Expression means the pericarp or peelings are pressed to squeeze out the oils. To retain valuable EOs, keep the lid on tight and store the bottles in a cool, dark place. Essential oils that we have kept for a long time have become more viscous. According to the Frontier Herbs Web site: "citrus oils deteriorate with age, patchouli and vetiver improve with age".

Essential oils generally have a long shelf-life, stored at room temperature away from direct light. Light and heat will deteriorate the oils. This is why we purchase essential oils that are bottled in dark glass and store them in a cool, dark place. We have never had an EO smell rancid. If this happens, discard it immediately. EOs will turn rancid if they are stored with water left over from the distillation process (see **hydrosols** and **distillates).** Commercial essential oils, manufactured under strictly controlled conditions, are usually dried over salts of sodium chloride to remove water before they are sold, to insure the longest possible shelf-life. When essential oils are diluted with a carrier or fixed oil, they can turn rancid. Any good-quality fixed oil will eventually turn rancid, especially when water, fresh plant material that contains moisture, or bacteria are introduced.

For aromatherapy and body products, be sure that you buy only pure essential oils and not synthetic fragrances. When adding essential oils to a product remember that they are chemically complex and concentrated. Use sparingly, and combine only a few at a time.

EOs contain literally hundreds of biochemicals, which can be used in many applications from household cleansers to aromatherapy to insect repellents or first aid. "The essential oil of oregano, for example, is twenty-six times more powerful as an antiseptic than phenol, which is the active ingredient in many commercial cleansing materials." From *The Complete Book of Essential Oils & Aromatherapy* by Valerie Ann Worwood.

To learn more about the chemistry of these oils, study books such as *The Big Book of Herbs* by Arthur Tucker and Thomas DeBaggio or enroll in the American College of Health Care Science in Portland, Oregon (www.achs.edu). James A. Duke, PhD created the Phytochemical Data Base online at http://www.ars-grin.gov/cgi-bin/duke, which contains a mind-boggling amount of scientific information on plants and their essential oils. Essential oil users should consider investing in the book, *Essential Oil Safety* by Tisserand & Balacs. We have many good books, articles, and Web sites listed in our **sources.**

EOs should not be applied or used neat on the body. Neat means straight; using the EO directly from the bottle to the skin. Most essential oils must be diluted in a carrier before being applied to the skin. Avoid essential oil contact with eyes, sensitive skin or mucous membranes. Always wash hands and surfaces after making products that contain essential oils. When making essential oil products and remedies, provide adequate ventilation in the room, wear chemical-resistant gloves and be aware that extended exposure may result in headache or nausea. Counteract these symptoms by drinking lots of water and getting to fresh air.

Use whole milk, mayonnaise or vegetable oil to dilute essential oil spills or accidental applications, then wash with soap and water. Many essential oils are solvents and will deteriorate plastics and finishes on furniture. EOs are flammable. Keep them away from open flames.

Caution: Keep essential oils away from the reach of children. Do not take essential oils internally or drop them into ears or eyes. Do not apply essential oils to babies or children without professional consultation. If you suffer from serious medical conditions, do not use essential oils without medical supervision. Pregnant and nursing women should consult with their health care providers before using essential oils and herbs.

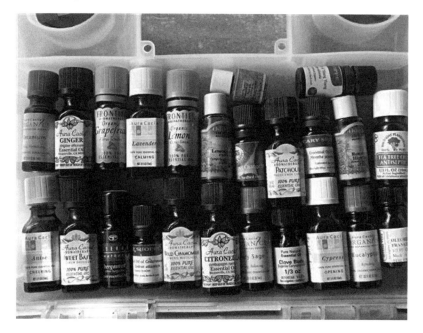

we use our collection of essential oils for aromatherapy, spa products, first aid and household cleaners

patch test

People have different sensitivities to plants and oils. If you have very sensitive skin or are taking prescription medication, it is prudent to do a "patch test" for every new essential oil before exposing larger areas of your body to the oil. Mix three drops of the essential oil to 1/2 teaspoon carrier oil. Apply this mixture to the pad of a Band-Aid® and secure the bandage to the inner part of the forearm. Leave on for 48 hours. If the area shows any irritation under or around the patch, the EO should not be used.

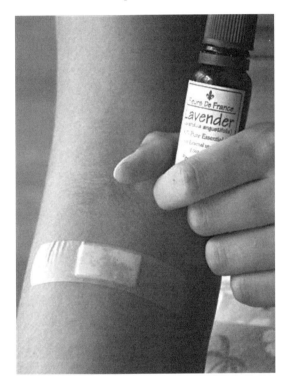

if you are new to essential oils or have allergies, we recommend doing a patch test

essential oils that we use most often in the creative herbal home

We use essential oils daily to relax, uplift, restore energy, relieve tension, keep healthy and ease the stress of travel. One you get to know the oils and become familiar with their fragrances and characteristics, you may find them an essential part of your life.

Basil (*Ocimum basilicum*)—uplifting, good for stress and indecisiveness, helps against mental fatigue; spicy and sweet scent with hint of anise. Some actions: antidepressant, antiseptic, anti-spasmodic, anti-venomous, aphrodisiac, bactericidal, insecticidal, nervine, prophylactic, restorative, stimulant. *Caution: Basil may cause an allergic reaction. Avoid basil oil during pregnancy.*

Bergamot (*Citrus bergamia, C. aurantium* subsp. *bergamia*)— refreshing and uplifting, balancing effect on emotions, warming; scent is clean and sweet, slight fruit and citrus. Some actions: antidepressant, anti-inflammatory, antiseptic, anti-spasmodic, carminative, deodorant, parasiticidal, vermifuge. *Caution: since this e.o. is high in bergapten, it is phototoxic in concentration, which means be careful in applying it to skin since it causes photosensitivity. Bergapten-free bergamot oils are now available.*

Cedarwood (*Cedrus species*)—soothing and harmonious, warming and sensual; pleasant woody fragrance with hint of camphor. Some actions: antiseptic, anti-putrescent, aphrodisiac, expectorant, fungicidal. *Caution: Do not use cedarwood during pregnancy.*

Chamomile, German (*Matricaria recutita*), syn. (*M. chamomilla*) —is good for skin care, gentle, soothing, warming and relaxing; strong sweet herby perfume. Use sparingly since it can be overwhelming or cloying in large amounts. Some actions: anti-allergenic, antidepressant, anti-inflammatory, antiseptic, bactericidal, emollient, fungicidal, nervine, sedative, vermifuge. German chamomile is also known as blue chamomile because the essential oil is deeply blue colored. This oil is the more costly of the two chamomile oils.

Chamomile, Roman (*Chamaemelum nobile*) —good for skin care, gentle, soothing, warming and relaxing; strong sweet herby fragrance with a hint of apples. Use sparingly, though not quite as heady as German chamomile. Some actions: analgesic, antidepressant, anti-inflammatory, antiseptic, bactericidal, digestive, emollient, hypnotic, nervine, sedative, vermifuge. *Caution: Care should be taken when ingesting or using this chamomile, since it may cause allergic responses in those with ragweed allergies.*

Citronella (*Cymbopogon nardus*) —stimulant, used more than any other essential oil as an insect repellent; bright and strong lemon perfume. Some actions: antiseptic, antioxidant, bactericidal, deodorant, fungicidal, insecticidal, sedative (to the nervous system) and stimulant. The monoterpenol, farnesol, contributes to the insecticidal properties of citronella. *Caution: Citronella may cause an allergic reaction.*

Clary Sage (*Salvia sclarea*) —warming, relaxing, uplifting, induces a sense of well being; sweet, heady herbal fragrance. The oil can be offensive to some. Some actions: anti-inflammatory, anti-microbial, anti-spasmodic, aphrodisiac, digestive, insecticidal, nervine, sedative. *Caution: Do not use clary sage during pregnancy.*

Clove (*Syzygium aromaticum*)—stimulating, helps with nervousness and mental fatigue, warming; clove bud perfume is strong spice, both hot and sweet. Some actions: anesthetic, antibiotic, anti-fungal, antiseptic, anti-viral, aphrodisiac, larvicidal, vermifuge. *Caution: Clove oil may cause an allergic reaction; the oil irritates mucous membranes and the skin. Do not use clove oil during pregnancy.*

Eucalyptus (*Eucalyptus globulus*)—head-clearing and cooling, good for muscular fatigue; big head-clearing scent that is pungent with camphor, slight pine-like resin. Some actions: analgesic, antiseptic, anti-viral, bactericidal, decongestant, deodorant, expectorant, insecticidal, parasiticidal, stimulant, vermifuge. Eucalyptus oil kills dust mites. It is important to note that eucalyptus oil is especially effective against the bacterial organism, *Staphylococcus* when used as an ingredient in cleaning agents. *Caution: Staph infections can be life threatening. Consult your health care provider immediately if staph symptoms are suspected. Eucalyptus causes violent allergic reactions in some people. Always dilute eucalyptus oil, as it can be a skin irritant. Do not use in cases of high blood pressure or epilepsy.*

Lavender (*Lavandula angustifolia*)—relaxing, soothing, uplifting and refreshing, blends well with other oils; its perfume is both floral and herby with barely a hint of balsam. Some actions: analgesic, antidepressant, anti-microbial, antiseptic, antitoxic, deodorant, insecticidal, nervine, restorative, sedative, stimulant, vermifuge. Lavandin (*Lavandula xintermedia)* has basically the same actions as *L. angustifolia*, though more obscure. It has much more camphor to the nose and works well for respiratory, muscular, deodorant and disinfectant purposes.

Lemon oil (*Citrus limon*)—increases the sense of well-being and is uplifting, brightens spirit; fragrance is sharp, clean, citrus. The EO is cold-pressed from the outer part of the fresh peel; limit to 10% in fragrance compounds. Some actions: anti-microbial, antioxidant, antiseptic, astringent, insecticidal, tonic, vermifuge. *Caution: Lemon oil may cause photosensitivity or an allergic reaction. Do not use lemon oil during pregnancy.*

Lemongrass (*Cymbopogon citratus*)—soothing and relaxing; the friendly herbal lemon fragrance of lemongrass makes it one of the top ten EOs sold for its perfume. Some actions: analgesic, antidepressant, anti-microbial, antioxidant, antiseptic, deodorant, fungicidal, insecticidal, nervine, sedative (nervous system), stimulant, tonic. Farnesol, a sesquiterpenol, contributes to the insecticidal properties of this essential oil. *Caution: Lemongrass may cause an allergic reaction or skin sensitivity; it must be diluted.*

Neroli (*Citrus aurantium* var. *amara*)—soothing, sensual, calms nerves, anxiety, and fear; the fragrance is exotic, floral and sweet, with a delicate spice note. This oil is made from a distillation of the fresh flowers and is sometimes sold as orange blossom oil. Some actions: antidepressant, antiseptic, aphrodisiac, deodorant, emollient, fungicidal, mild hypnotic, nerve stimulant. Although it is citrus, the EO. from the blossom does not seem to be phototoxic or irritating. Petitgrain was originally made from the fruit of this plant, today it is often made from the leaves and peels. It is stronger and sharper than neroli, but has some of the same attributes. *Caution: petitgrain can be allergenic.*

Oregano (*Origanum vulgare*)—sometimes listed as *Thymus capitatus,* which is a species of thyme; stimulating, with a strong, hot, medicinal herb smell. Some actions: strong antiseptic, antiviral, bactericidal, expectorant, fungicidal, parasiticidal, stimulant. *Caution: Both sources of oregano oil cause burning and are extremely irritating to mucous membranes and inflamed tissue when applied undiluted or in strong dilution. Oregano oil may cause an allergic reaction. Do not use during pregnancy.*

Patchouli (*Pogostemon cablin*), syn. (*P. patchouli*)—relaxing, helps relieve stress and nerves; the scent is heavy and deep, earthy and musty, resinous and unmistakable. Some actions: antidepressant, anti-microbial, antiseptic, antitoxic, anti-viral, aphrodisiac, deodorant, fungicidal, insecticidal, sedative in small amounts, stimulant in large amounts. It has a tendency to be overwhelming, if you wear it too heavily.

Pennyroyal (*Mentha pulegium*)—scent is strong, a combination of mint and oregano. Some actions: antiseptic, insect repellent and stimulant. The essential oil is still marketed as a flea repellent despite reports of severe reactions and death of pets associated with its use. *Caution: This oil should never be taken internally as it can cause death due to its high content of pulegone; some authorities discourage its use completely. Do not use pennyroyal oil on cats or dogs. Never use pennyroyal during pregnancy. Keep this and all essential oils out of the reach of children.*

Peppermint (*Mentha xpiperita*)—warming, stimulating, helps to clear the head and improve focus; strong, bright mint and peppery aroma. Some actions: anti-inflammatory, anti-microbial, antiseptic, decongestant, digestive, expectorant, insect repellent, nervine, vermifuge. The phenol, menthol comprises the largest percentage of the EO, with smaller amounts of menthyl acetate, menthone, cineol, pinene and limonene *Caution: In large amounts, the oil can cause irritation to the mucous membranes. Some people may have allergic reactions to peppermint oil. Peppermint should not be given to babies in any form.*

Rose geranium (*Pelargonium graveolens*)—relaxing, soothing, and balancing, often helps to lessen stress and anxiety; the fragrance is rose first, followed by a herbaceous note, and sometimes a bit of citrus depending upon the origin of the essential oil. Some actions: antidepressant, anti-inflammatory, antiseptic, astringent, deodorant, fungicidal, insecticidal, tonic, vermifuge. The oil is comprised of varying percentages of geranic acid; the alcohols geraniol, citronellol, linalool, myrtenol, terpineol; the aldehyde, citrol; the ketone, menthone and the phenol, eugenol. *Caution: Large quantities of the oil may cause skin irritation or sensitivity in some individuals.*

Rosemary (*Rosmarinus officinalis*)—refreshing, stimulating, and uplifting, balancing effect on emotions and is warming; the aroma is piney and resinous, with a bit of camphor, and sometimes an afterthought of citrus. A strong stimulant, it can be used as a steam inhalation to stimulate the mind or loosen congestion, for poor circulation, or used in liniments to relieve muscular aches. Some actions: antidepressant, anti-microbial, antioxidant, antiseptic, aphrodisiac, digestive, fungicidal, nervine, paraciticide, restorative, stimulant. Rosemary EO contains the alcohol, borneol; the aldehyde, cuminic; the ester, bornyl acetate; the ketones camphor and cineol; the sesquiterpene, caryophyllene and the terpenes, camphene and pinene. *Caution: Avoid rosemary oil if you are pregnant, have epilepsy or high blood pressure. Avoid applying the oil on or around varicose veins.*

Sandalwood (*Santalum album*)—relaxing, warming, grounding, and sensual; its exotic perfume is a warm combination of wood and spice with a touch of balsam. Some actions: antidepressant, antiseptic, aphrodisiac, bactericidal, emollient, fungicidal, insecticidal, sedative.

Sweet orange (*Citrus sinensis*)—relaxing and balancing, the fragrance of this essential oil, which is extracted from the fresh peel, is light and sweet, fruity with bright citrus. Some actions: antidepressant, anti-inflammatory, antiseptic, bactericidal, fungicidal and insect repellent. *Caution: Orange oil may cause photosensitivity or allergic reaction. Do not wear orange oil on skin exposed to sunlight or tanning lights.*

Tangerine (*Citrus reticulata*), sometimes referred to as **Mandarin**—relaxing and cheering; a lively, sweet citrus fragrance that is a bit lighter than orange (*C. sinensis*). Some actions: antiseptic, anti-spasmodic, calmative, digestive, mild sedative. *Caution: May cause photosensitivity. Do not wear citrus oils on skin exposed to sunlight or tanning lights.*

Tea tree (*Melaleuca alternifolia*)—head-clearing and powerful; strong medicinal odor with similarities to both eucalyptus and camphor. Tea tree has the amazing ability to combat bacteria, fungi and viruses. Some actions: antibiotic, anti-inflammatory, antiseptic, anti-viral, bactericidal, fungicidal, immuno-stimulant, insecticidal, parasiticidal.

Thyme (*Thymus vulgaris*)—strong and stabilizing; all thymes have a powerful herbal scent—red thyme is warm and stronger of spice while white thyme is milder and has a slight sweetness. Some actions: anti-microbial, antioxidant, antiseptic, astringent, aphrodisiac, nervine, stimulant, tonic and vermifuge. Red thyme oil has not been distilled again, so it is the crude distillate, retaining its red color; it is stronger than distilled thyme. White thyme has been distilled twice, which makes it a clear oil; it is not as strong as red thyme and therefore less irritating. *Caution: Thyme oils are extremely irritating to inflamed tissue and mucous membranes. Always use thyme in dilution. Do not use thyme if pregnant, nursing or if you have high blood pressure.*

Ylang-ylang (*Cananga odorata*)—soothing, warming and sensual, stabilizes emotions; heady floral, sweet perfume, may be overwhelming and offensive to sensitive individuals; use in small amounts. Some actions: antidepressant, anti-infectious, antiseptic, aphrodisiac, nervine, tonic, sedative to the nervous system, and stimulant to circulatory system. *Caution: Avoid using ylang-ylang on inflamed skin. Overuse of the oil can induce headache or nausea.*

Vetiver (*Vetiveria zizanoides*)—relaxing, uplifting and warming, a sensual, comforting tonic; this root distillate has a deep, dark earthy scent with a hint of sweet and smoke. Often used as a fixative and in bath products for men. Some actions: antiseptic, aphrodisiac, insect repellent, sedative for nervous system, stimulant for circulatory system, vermifuge.

antiseptic essential oils

Virtually all essential oils are antiseptic, some more than others. We use them in our household preparations because they destroy and help to prevent the growth of microbes.

Basil (*avoid during pregnancy and nursing*)
Citronella (*may cause allergic reaction*)
Chamomile (*may cause dermatitis*)
Clove (*may cause irritation to skin or mucous membranes*)
Eucalyptus (*avoid during pregnancy and nursing*)
Geranium
Lavender
Lemongrass (*may cause irritation of skin*)
Marjoram (*avoid during pregnancy and nursing*)
Neroli
Oregano (*avoid during pregnancy and nursing, may cause irritation to skin or mucous membranes*)
Patchouli
Peppermint
Rosemary (*avoid during pregnancy and nursing; do not use if you have high blood pressure or epilepsy*)
Sandalwood
Sweet Orange (*may cause photosensitivity*)
Tea tree
Thyme (*avoid during pregnancy and nursing; do not use if you have high blood pressure; some thymes have toxic amounts of phenols such as carvacrol and thymol, so use carefully*)
Vetiver
Ylang-ylang (*may cause nausea or headaches in sensitive individuals*)

insect-repellent essential oils

These oils, in random combination seem to be effective against mosquitoes, gnats, chiggers, biting flies and moths that lay eggs on wool. They have not been effective against "no-see-'ems," moths that are attracted to lights at night, spiders or ticks.

Essential oils are volatile by nature. This means that they evaporate quickly and must be reapplied regularly to work. *Caution: It is safer to use citrus oils in repellent agents that will not be applied to the skin, since studies show that they can cause phototoxicity. We tend not to use citrus oils in skin preparations, but use them often in and around the house.*

Catnip
Cedarwood (*do not use during pregnancy and nursing*)
Citronella (*may cause allergic reaction*)
Eucalyptus (*may cause allergic reactions*)
Lavender
Lemon (*may cause photosensitivity*)
Lemon balm
Lemongrass (*may cause irritation of skin*)
Patchouli
Peppermint (*do not give peppermint, in any form, to babies*)
Rose geranium
Sandalwood
Sweet orange (*may cause photosensitivity*)
Vetiver

nervine and sedative essential oils

Caution: Avoid driving or operating machinery after a relaxing massage or other treatment using soporific or sedative EOs.

Chamomile, **German** and **Roman** (*may cause dermatitis*)
Clary sage (*avoid during pregnancy and nursing; do not use when drinking alcohol*)
Lavender
Sandalwood
Tangerine (*may cause photosensitivity or dermatological reaction*)

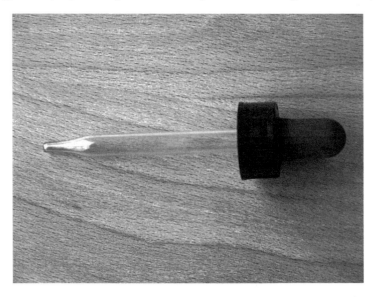

use glass droppers to measure EOs

estimated measurement by drops
1 dropperful = about 35 drops or 1/4 teaspoon
2 1/2 droppersful = about 87 drops or 1/2 teaspoon
5 droppersful = about 175 drops or 1 teaspoon

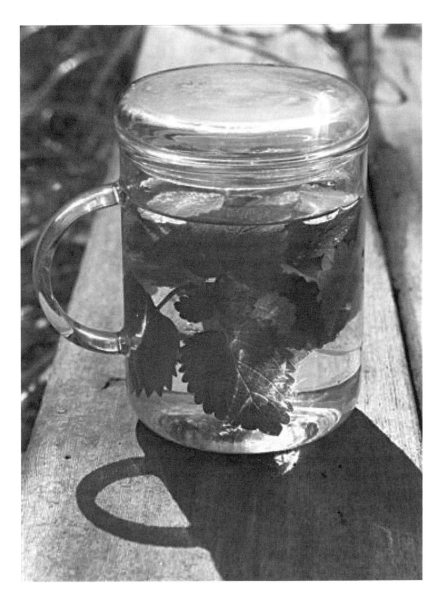

infusion of lemon balm

infusions and decoctions

The following list of definitions is from *Webster's Third New International Dictionary*. Springfield, Massachusetts: G. & C. Merriam Company.

decoction—"the act or process of boiling, usually in water, so as to extract the flavor or active principle; a liquid preparation made by boiling a medicinal plant with water, usually in the proportion of 5 parts medicinal drug to 100 part water."

infusion—"the steeping or soaking, usually in water, of a substance (as a plant drug) in order to extract its virtues."

shrub—"a beverage made by adding acidulated fruit juice to iced water."

simple—"a plant used for its supposed medicinal properties; a vegetable drug or medicinal preparation having only one ingredient."

suspension—"the state of a substance when its particles are mixed with but undissolved in a fluid or solid."

syrup—"a thick sticky liquid consisting of a concentrated solution of sugar and water with or without the addition of a flavoring agent or medicinal substance."

tea—"an aromatic beverage that is prepared from cured tea leaves (*Camellia sinensis*) by infusion with boiling water and has mild stimulant and tonic properties due to the alkaloid caffeine and is capable of being strongly astringent from the presence of tannin; any of numerous plants somewhat resembling tea in appearance or properties; an infusion prepared from their leaves and used medicinally or as a beverage, used usually with qualifying adjective or attribute (i.e.: sage tea, mint tea)."

tisane—"an infusion usually of dried leaves or flowers that is used for a beverage or for mildly medicinal effects."

Generally, the term tea refers to beverages made from the leaves of the tea plant *Camellia sinensis*. **Infusion** is the proper term for beverages made from herbs; however, **herb tea** and herbal infusion are used interchangeably nowadays. Both **simple** and **tisane** are words, used in the past, quite simply to describe a tea or infusion made with herbs, usually a single herb rather than a combination.

An **infusion** is the maceration of leaves or flowers, in a liquid which is most often water, but can be juice, milk, cream, vinegar, alcohol, etc., in order to extract its flavor or active principles. Infusion methods include maceration, percolation, digestion, and dilution of extracts. As in a hot herbal infusion, water is heated barely to a boil, leaves and/or flowers are dropped in, the pan is covered and the herbs are allowed to infuse for anywhere from three to ten minutes. The infusion can then be strained and drunk hot, or it can be cooled to room temperature and then used. It is best to use the infusion on the day it is prepared, otherwise refrigerate it after it has cooled to room temperature and use it within 24 hours. Cold water infusions can also be prepared; however, it takes longer to extract the active principles. Keep refrigerated and use within two days of preparation. Given below are recipes for both cold and hot infusions, herb vinegar, herbal syrups and shrubs. For preparing an infusion using alcohol, please see our **tincture** chapter.

A **decoction** is almost always made with water. Decoctions are often made with the harder parts of plants such as root, bark or berries, rather than leaves or flowers, and generally the water is boiled. The medicinal plants are usually tough roots, barks and hard seeds that will not yield active constituents to cooler temperatures. The cooking time varies depending on the plant material; it is generally about 15 minutes to an hour. Decoctions can be taken hot, warm, or at room temperature. Once cooled, refrigerate and use within 24 hours.

Herbs that should not be prepared by decoction include members of the mint family and other families valued for their essential oils because the volatile oils would be lost in the steam. Comfrey, senna and slippery elm contain mucilage that is rendered useless in boiling water. If these plants are to be used with herbs in a formula, the plants may be added to the solution after it has been removed from the heat. We have two decoction methods below—one is a boiled one and the other is an overnight extraction.

Medicinal **syrups** are often prepared with sugar or honey, usually at a proportion of two parts sugar or honey to one part liquid, or sometimes in equal parts. The liquid is usually an herbal concentrate—herbs that are infused—and then reduced by simmering so that the water evaporates and the liquid thickens. The sweetener helps to preserve the herbal extract. Sometimes a little alcohol, such as brandy is added also to aid in preserving.

Syrup has the advantage of being sticky which helps the medicine adhere to tissues longer than an infusion made with water. Syrup is the usual menstruum for cough remedies. "Just a spoonful of sugar helps the medicine go down," however sometimes a sick person may not be able to tolerate the sweet flavor but can sip an herbal infusion. We also use syrups for beverages and in recipes— for these we tend to use less sweetener and more water—therefore they are less concentrated and are of a thinner consistency. Using honey or maple syrup are both natural ways of sweetening a syrup. If you are looking for strong herbal flavor, both of the aforementioned liquid sweeteners have their own dominant taste, which will affect the flavor of the syrup. Stevia leaves can be used to sweeten an infusion, however, they do not thicken or become syrupy like honey or sugar. All syrups should be kept in the refrigerator. Shrub is a kind of syrup; however, it is prepared with vinegar or alcohol.

It is important to use good water to prepare the most healthful herbal infusions and decoctions. If the water from your faucet is chlorinated or chemically treated, we recommend buying spring water or obtaining it from a more natural source.

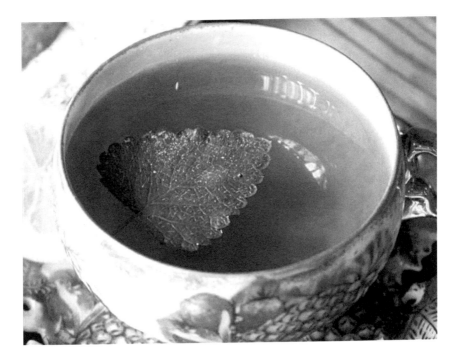

a lovely cup of tea with lemon balm

herbal infusion or herb tea

Fresh or dried, herbs that we use most often for infusions are orange mint, lemon balm or verbena, bee balm, common sage and pineapple sage, spearmint, peppermint, and chamomile flowers. We also like rosehips, raspberry leaf, red clover, corn silk, linden, milky oats, lemongrass, stevia and lemon or cinnamon basil. Of course, there are many more, but those listed are the ones that we use most often. Sometimes we prepare an herb infusion with just a single herb or flower. However, oftentimes we use a combination of two or three herbs to make a synergistic blend. To prepare just 1 or 2 cups, quarter or halve the recipe below.

Makes about 1 quart

1 quart water
Generous 2 cups packed fresh herb leaves and flowers

Rinse the herbs if they are dirty and pat or spin them dry. Bring the water just barely to a boil in a non-reactive saucepan and then remove from heat. Add the herb leaves and cover. For a hot beverage, steep for about 5 minutes, taste it for desired strength and serve, or let steep for a few minutes more. Otherwise, let steep for about 30 minutes, or until the infusion is room temperature. Keep in mind, the longer the herb is infused, the more starches and tannins will be extracted from the herb into the solution.

To prepare cold infusions or ice cubes: Strain the herbs and pour the infusion into a glass jar or pitcher and refrigerate and use within 24 to 48 hours. Or pour the infusion into ice cube trays and freeze until hard. Once frozen, pop the cubes into freezer, zip-close bags and label. Be sure to label, because all of the ice cubes tend to look alike once frozen and you won't be able to tell them apart.

sun tea, overnight or refrigerator infusions

The concept of these infusions is to allow the sun or the moon, or just the water, to infuse with the herbs for a longer period of time to extract the flavor and medicine of the herbs. For sun tea the jar is set out in the sun, preferably in the herb garden, and the heat of the sun warms the water and helps to extract the herbal goodness from the herbs—you can leave the infusion out for 2 to 8 hours—the longer the time, the stronger the infusion. Once infused, strain the herbs from the infusion and refrigerate; use within 24 to 48 hours.

For a lunar tea or infusion, which we especially like to do for a full moon tea (although all phases are agreeable!) we gather the herbs before dusk and place them in a jar with cold water, which we set out in a chosen place in the garden and let the moon rays do their magic overnight. Preparing an overnight infusion of herbs and cold water and leaving it on the kitchen counter or placing it in the refrigerator is also perfectly acceptable—anywhere we put them is fine—as long as we do it with good intent. Cold infusions are a good way for kids to make mint tea because there is no heating required.

You may easily halve or double this recipe.

Makes about 1/2 gallon

1/2 gallon water
About 4 cups packed fresh herb leaves and flowers

Rinse the herbs if they are dirty and pat them dry. Place them in a large clean jar or crock that you reserve for this purpose. Pour the water over the herbs and stir if desired, though it is not necessary.

Cover with cheesecloth or muslin and secure, or use a lid, and place in the garden. Say a blessing if you desire. If making a sun tea, leave for a few hours or all day. Leave overnight for a moon tea.

These infusions will be milder in flavor than a hot infusion, but they will be magical. You can either strain the herbs from the tea or leave them; store in a cool place for a day or in the refrigerator for 24 to 48 hours. It is best to drink an infusion in the first 24 hours.

overnight extraction

Overnight infusions are thought to be a better remedy from roots when they are lightly decocted, rather than boiling them for a long time. Medicinal roots such as burdock and dandelion contain albumen and are softened with heat first and then the medicinal properties are extracted with the help of time and plant enzymes as in this overnight recipe. As with all preparations made with only water, refrigerate and use within 24 to 48 hours.

Makes 1 quart

About 1/2 cup of root, bark, berries, or other plant parts chopped into small pieces or ground into powder
1 quart of just-boiled water

Place the clean herb plant parts in a clean quart jar. Pour the boiling water, cover, and let stand overnight. Strain off, refrigerate and use as needed in 24 to 48 hours.

decoctions and suspensions

We decided to show you one of the best and easiest ways of making a decoction.

> *"Soup, soup, beautiful soup!"*
> --Lewis Carroll

delicious & good-for-you winter soup with astragalus root

Here is a powerful soup to jumpstart your immune system and warm your core. Decocting the astragalus root in the soup is a simple way to slip the benefits of this medicinal root into your loved ones' bowls and they will never know. Except for the bay leaf and astragalus, all of the ingredients can be regarded as suspensions because the foods and seasonings are medicinally nutritious and they are eaten with the decoction broth.

The astragalus root and shiitake are believed to boost the immune system. The bay leaf, because it is fresh, gives the soup a hint of citrus and spice. Remove the astragalus root or bay leaf when you ladle out the soup. The ginger and chiles will warm you. The garlic is a cure-all for many illnesses. The tofu is the only vegetable source of a complete protein plus it is a phytoestrogen.

Of course there are infinite variations that can be made here—use what you have on hand or whatever you like best—be innovative—just be sure to use the astragalus and garlic. You can use vegetable stock in place of the water and miso.

Makes 2 to 4 servings

Handful dried shiitake mushrooms, stems removed, broken or
chopped coarsely
1 cup nearly boiling water
2 to 3 tablespoons extra-virgin olive oil
1 medium onion, peeled and chopped
1 large sweet potato, peeled, sliced and diced
2-inch piece gingerroot, peeled and chopped fine
1 whole bulb garlic, peeled and chopped
About 12-ounces firm tofu cut into 3/4-inch cubes
1 quart water
1 stick astragalus root, broken in half
2 bay leaves
2 small dried chiles, stemmed and seeded, chopped coarsely
1 bunch of greens (about 2 packed cups cut into chiffonade)—
we like kale, chard, dandelion, spinach, arugula, cress, mustard,
collard or any combination thereof
1 generous teaspoon dried oregano leaves, crumbled
About 3 tablespoons miso, mellow yellow or red
Sea salt

Put the shiitake into a small bowl and pour the cup of hot water on
them; let stand.

Heat the oil in a large, heavy-bottomed soup pot or Dutch oven
over medium heat. Add the onion and stir for about 3 minutes. Add
the sweet potato, stir and cover for another minute or two. Add
the gingerroot, garlic and tofu, stir well, cover and cook for 2 to 3
minutes.

Add the water, astragalus root, bay leaves and chiles, stir well,
cover and bring to a simmer. Reduce heat so soup is barely
simmering, and cook for 10 to 15 minutes.

Ladle about 1/2 cup of the soup broth into a bowl. Stir the rehydrated shiitake with the mushroom liqueur, greens and oregano and about 1 teaspoon salt into the soup pot and cover. Put the miso paste into the bowl with the hot soup broth and stir with a fork until dissolved. Add this to the soup pot and stir. The soup should be just below simmering since boiling miso will diminish its nutritional value.

Cook until the greens are tender and carefully taste for seasoning and adjust with salt if necessary. Cover and let sit until ready to serve.

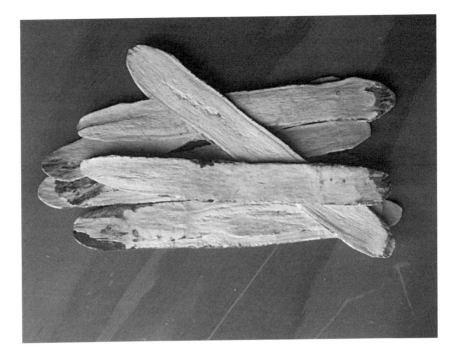

astragalus root

herbal vinegars

Preparing herbal-infused vinegars is a pleasure for the herb gardener, yielding a simple way to concentrate herb flavor and store it for the year. Brightly-colored bottles of opal basil vinegar and tarragon vinegar are two summer traditions that we consider as kitchen essentials. They enhance salads and sauces all throughout the year. Part of the fun of making vinegars is experimenting with different herbs. Often a combination of two or three herbs offers a pleasant surprise. The rewards are worth the little amount of effort it takes to make herbal vinegars.

Organic apple cider vinegar, good quality rice and white wine vinegars, make the best herb vinegars. We often use organic apple cider vinegar—the flavor works well with the flavor of many herbs—but it doesn't give the clean bright colors as clear vinegar does. We also like to use organic brown rice vinegar, and *umeboshi* plum vinegar (sometimes called *ume*) for small batches and special blends. The latter is very salty—the plums are salted and fermented before being made into vinegar—so taste before deciding to make herbal vinegar with this.

Balsamic and red wine vinegar are very strong; the flavors of the herbs do not shine through as well so we generally don't make herb vinegars with them. Some people prefer the robust herbs such as oregano, rosemary or even chiles with red wine vinegar. We like a sherry vinegar with serranos or jalapenos as a garnish for our black bean soup. Experiment if this appeals to you.

We do not use distilled vinegar—except for cleaning house—it is too harsh for the flavor of most herbs. According to *The New Whole Foods Encyclopedia*, in reference to distilled vinegar, author Rebecca Wood states, "It may be synthetic ethanol made by direct chemical oxidation of wood or fossil fuels. Distilled and other highly processed vinegars are mineral deficient, and when consumed, pull calcium and other minerals from the bones and tissues."

Homemade vinegar should not be used unless the acid level is between 4 to 6 % and it has been pasteurized. Vinegar owes its preservative qualities to the mild acetic acid content. Do not add water to flavored vinegars as this would dilute the acid. Be sure to cover the herb completely with vinegar to avoid the growth of mold. Discard any moldy vinegar. Vinegar that develops a "mother" or becomes ropy and cloudy can be strained, brought to a boil and rebottled. Store vinegars, tightly capped, in a cool dark place. Label contents in bottle.

Note: When adding fresh fruit such as raspberries, blueberries, or peaches to vinegar, it is best to bring the vinegar to a simmer, stir in the washed fruit, and sugar if you are using it, and let cool. Proceed as described with the directions for infusing herbal vinegar.

Tip: After we have had vinegars sit around for more than a year or so, rather than discard them, we generally relegate them to washing salads.

basic herb vinegar

Some good choices of herbs for making vinegars are: anise hyssop, basil, especially the purple varieties; chile peppers; chive with chive blossoms; dill; garlic; lavender; all of the lemon herbs; lovage; marigold; mint; nasturtium flowers, oregano; rosemary; sage; savory and tarragon. For smaller amounts, this recipe is easily halved.

Makes 1 quart

About 1 quart vinegar
2 to 3 cups loosely packed herbs and/or flowers

Harvest your herbs on a sunny morning, clean the sprigs if necessary and pat them dry. Bruise them slightly. Fill clean jars about half to three-quarters full of the herbs you have chosen and cover them with vinegar. Use plastic rather than metal lids, or before you screw on the lid, cover the mouth of the jar with a double-layer of plastic wrap. (The plastic wrap fix is for the short term only. Eventually the acid of the vinegar leaches out and corrodes metal lids, so we recommend buying the plastic lids to fit the canning jars.) Label the jars.

There are a few different ways to infuse the herbs and vinegar. The herbs begin to flavor the vinegar in just a few hours. However, generally the best flavor is achieved by infusing the herbs for a few weeks. We've seen recipes that recommend two weeks and some say up to six weeks. We suggest that you taste your herb vinegar infusion once a week until you are happy with the flavor.

The other conundrum is whether to place the vinegar in the sunlight or in a dark place. For years, Susan has followed the process that she first learned, by setting the jars out in the herb garden and letting the sun do its work to infuse the herbs and vinegar. Tina steeps her vinegars in a dark place. Since we have learned that light deteriorates essential oils, Susan did an experiment of making herbal vinegar with the exact same proportions of herb to vinegar. At the same time she put one in the sun and one in the cool, dark pantry. After four weeks time, the vinegars looked similar in color, however, the herb that was in the sun had deteriorated much more—it was more slimy in texture. Upon tasting, the sun infusion was stronger, bitter-tasting and more acidic. The infusion kept in the dark had a bit milder flavor, though was plenty flavorful, was all-around better tasting and was not nearly as bitter or acidic. Thus, we agree with the herbalists who recommend that the infusions should be steeped in a cool, dark place and shaken daily.

When you begin steeping herbs in vinegar in the morning, it can be used that evening since it will begin flavoring the vinegar immediately. The longer it stands—the more flavor it will have. At a certain point, it will begin to change taste. The herbs will deteriorate and the flavor will not be as bright. A general rule of thumb for infusion is about 2 to 4 weeks. We recommend that you taste your vinegar in about 10 days to 2 weeks time and see if you are happy with the flavor; taste every few days or once a week thereafter until you have achieved the flavor that you are seeking.

Whichever method you choose to infuse—light or dark—after the allotted time the herbs will need to be removed. Open the jars, and pour the vinegar through a strainer to remove the herbs. Using a funnel, pour the vinegar into smaller bottles and label. Store the vinegars in a cool, dark place and use them within a year.

herb combinations used for making flavored vinegar

We also like to make some blends of herbs for tasty vinegars. A general rule of thumb is never to combine more than two or three herbs in a vinegar because the flavors become muddy. Be creative and combine some of your favorite herbs and flowers!
Here are 4 favorite combinations:

chive, dill & nasturtium flowers
Apple cider, rice or white wine vinegar
Chives
Dill sprigs
Orange, red, or mahogany nasturtiums

lemon, ginger & lemon herbs
Rice or white wine vinegar
Lemon slices, seeds removed
Thinly sliced gingerroot
Lemon balm, lemon basil, lemongrass, verbena, &/or lemon thyme

chiles, southwest herbs, & garlic
Apple cider, rice or white wine vinegar
Red or green chiles, pierced
Garlic cloves, peeled
Oregano, sage, thyme and/or mint

raspberry, vanilla, & orange mint
Rice or white wine vinegar
1 pint raspberries
1 vanilla bean
Orange mint or bergamot
2 tablespoons sugar, optional

herb syrups

Herb syrups are wonderful flavor essences that are good on all kinds of fruits and used in beverages. You can enjoy the health benefits of herbs while using them to sweeten tea and to make natural sodas. They can be added in place of the liquid in cakes, pie filling and sorbet. Brush the syrups on pound cakes, cupcakes, muffins or breads just out of the oven.

Although we have been making rose, violet, mint, ginger, and vanilla syrups for years, the inspiration for expanding our herbal horizon of syrups came from *The Herb Farm Cookbook* by Jerry Traunfeld, Scribner, 2000. He has many wonderful recipes using herbs syrups and cream infusions. Make these when you have fresh herbs or edible flowers in abundance, their flavor and aroma will bring a brightness to fruits, fruit salad and desserts.

For a medium syrup, equal parts of water and sugar are used. We do play around with the amount of sugar in this recipe. This recipe makes a sweet syrup. Depending upon what we are using the syrup for, we often cut the sugar back to 3/4 or 1 cup. For instance, when we make ginger syrup for ginger ale or a punch that has already sweet ingredients like pineapple juice, we use the lesser amount of sugar. Syrups can also be sweetened with maple syrup or honey, however their flavor will be dominate and lessen the flavor of the herbs.

basic herb syrup

Makes about 2 cups

1 1/2 cups water
1 1/2 cups sugar
About 8 to 10 herb sprigs or a large handful of leaves

To make a herb syrup, combine the water and sugar in a small saucepan. Place over moderate heat and bring to a boil; stir to dissolve sugar. Add the herbs bruising the leaves against the side of the pan with a spoon. Cover, remove from heat and let stand for at least 30 minutes.

Remove the leaves and squeeze them into the syrup to extract their flavor. Pour into a clean bottle or jar and label. This syrup can be made ahead and kept in the refrigerator for about 4 weeks.

If you want to keep the syrups for a long period of time, pour them into jars or bottles leaving at least an inch of headspace, place on the lid or cap, and label. We freeze them for up to one year. Remove from freezer the night before using and allow to thaw; or place the bottle in a bowl of warm (not hot) water to thaw more quickly. It is okay to thaw some, use what you need, and refreeze the syrup.

herbs and flowers used for making syrups

The following amounts are based on the recipe above yielding
approximately 2 cups of syrup. Amounts of herbs and herb flowers
used will vary and depend on the flavor of each individual herb, the
list below is for sprigs about 4 or 5 inches long. Be creative and try
your favorite herb or perhaps a combination of two.

Anise hyssop—6 to 8 sprigs with flowers, or a handful of flowers
Basil—6 to 8 sprigs of anise, cinnamon, green or lemon basil
Bay—10 to 12 fresh leaves
Chamomile—a generous handful
Elder flowers—3 or 4 large blooms
Ginger—about 1/4 to 1/3 cup thin slices of the root
Lavender—10 flower spikes or 1 tablespoon flowers
Lemon balm, lemon thyme, or lemon verbena—8 to 10 sprigs
Monarda—10 or 12 leaves, especially the petals of 2 or 3 blooms
Mint—10 to 12 sprigs of orange mint, peppermint or spearmint
Rose petals—about a handful (taste for flavor before using)
Rosemary—5 or 6 sprigs
Sage—4 common sage sprigs; 6 fruit-scented or pineapple sage
sprigs
Scented geraniums—12 to 15 leaves rose, nutmeg, lemon, coconut,
apple, ginger, etc.
Tarragon or Mexican tarragon—6 to 8 sprigs
Vanilla—1 bean, halved and split lengthwise
Violets—about 1 cup fresh-picked flowers
Herb seeds—about 1 tablespoon bruised anise, coriander or fennel
seeds (slightly green are best)

elderberry shrub with honey

We have been preparing elderberry shrub for years with only beneficial effects. Recently we found out that elderberries should always be cooked before being eaten to avoid ingesting unripe berries. Unripe berries contain prussic acid that causes cyanide poisoning if the berries are not cooked first before being consumed. (Brinker, 2000 www.herbalsafety.utep.edu/herbs). In the past, we made shrub without cooking the berries and believe that the vinegar "cooks" them. However, to be safe, we recommend that you bring your vinegar to a simmer, add the berries, remove from heat, then proceed with the recipe.

Recipes for shrubs vary greatly and date as far back as pre-colonial times. Shrubs can be made with sweetened fruit juice, fruit, vinegar, honey or sugar. Some suggest adding spirits such as rum or brandy to the shrub. We have never used spirits to make our shrubs but find the idea seductive.

Generally, shrubs are sipped from a cordial glass, poured over ice or served with a bit of sparkling water. They are a wonderful remedy for congestion and sore throat, and make an excellent tonic for the body. They tend to make us perspire when we drink them. We choose elderberries for this shrub, however; you may substitute other berries such as blueberries, raspberries, blackberries, currants, gooseberries or a combination thereof.

The recipe can easily be halved or quartered to make a smaller amount.

Makes about 2 quarts

2 cups elderberries
1 quart apple cider vinegar
1 quart honey

Wash and pick over the berries. Put the berries in a non-reactive pan. Pour the vinegar over the berries, cover and bring to a low simmer. Remove from heat and let stand overnight or up to two weeks in the refrigerator.

Mash the fruit vinegar and strain through cheesecloth or muslin. Add the honey and blend well. Bottle in dark glass, sterilized jars with non-metal lids and label. Keep out of reach of children.

Store in a cool dark place. We have never known of shrub to go bad in storage. However, it will do the body more good if it is used rather than stored. Use it within one year.

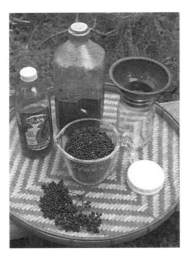

ingredients for making elderberry shrub

marion's habanero shrub

Our friend Marion Spear is the queen of shrubs. She makes them from all kinds of fruits and introduced us to chile pepper shrub. Yeehaw! Besides as a sipping beverage to clear the throat before singing, she uses them on ice cream, as a beverage with cream (rather like a syllabub), with whipped cream as a pie filling and in a multitude of other ways. If you can tolerate foods that have the characteristic capsaicin burn, you will find this shrub an invigorating, delicious tonic. The honey balances and subdues the heat without totally extinguishing it.

1/4 cup ripe, blemish-free habanero peppers
1 cup apple cider vinegar
Less than 1 cup honey

Wearing rubber gloves, wash and cut slits in the habaneros. Put the chiles in a sterilized pint-size jar and pour in the vinegar. Cover tightly. Place jar in the refrigerator for one week, or more.

After the vinegar has been infused with the flavor and heat of the habaneros, strain out the chiles. (Marion says not to discard these pickled peppers! Cover them with fresh vinegar or cook them up into a hot sauce.) Measure the habanero vinegar and stir in an equal measure of honey.

Label and store in a sterilized jar or bottle; keep out of reach of children.

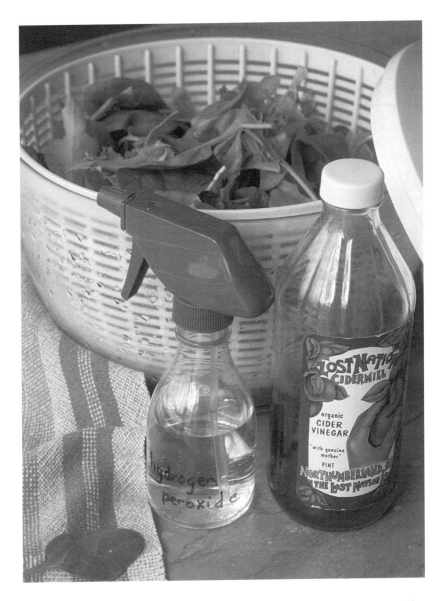

washing salad greens with vinegar and hydrogen peroxide

household preparations

*Because people have differing sensitivities to herbs and essential oils, do a **patch test** for allergies (see **definitions of terms** for instructions) before applying new substances to your body or environment.*

Housekeeping is a necessary nuisance for dedicated gardeners. All we really want to do is spend every waking moment planting and tending the garden. During the growing season, the house is just a place to write, sleep, eat and clean up.

Combating bugs, dirt and microbes is a never-ending process. To take care of the earth while defending our boundaries, we engage an arsenal of herbs, anti-bacterial and insect repellent essential oils, water, vinegar, baking soda, alcohol, hydrogen peroxide, surfactants and castile soap. **Ingredients** are listed in a separate chapter for easy reference.

We both get our water from wells and the electricity to pump the water is an expense; ground water is limited. Therefore, every drop is precious to the garden. From spring until early winter, house cleaning is a study in conservation. We prepare wash and rinse water with biodegradable ingredients in basins or buckets so that the gray water can be carried out to thirsty plants. (Of course, we let the hot wash and rinse water cool to room temperature before watering plants with them.)

For everyday washing, we choose a surfactant that is non-polluting and makes water "wetter." The manufacturer keeps the formula a secret; however, the chemistry can be understood. The compound is made up of molecules that are opposites, some are hydrophobic (don't like water) and the others are attracted to water. When the surfactant is mixed with water, the hydrophobic molecules try to separate from the water and the others stay. This action breaks the surface tension of water so that it does not bead up on surfaces — rather it flows into the crevices and around particles with ease, suspending them in solution. In the garden, the surfactant helps water flow between soil particles instead of beading up and running off the surface.

Castile soap is alkaline and most "dirt" that we are removing has an acid pH. Cooking oil and grease, garden soil and much of the food left on plates is acid-based and is broken up into smaller particles, lifted from the surface into the water and is floated away. Those of us with "hard" water (containing calcium, magnesium and/or sulfur) end up with soap scum in the sink and bathtub when we use soap.

For rinsing, vinegar is added to slightly acidify the water. This cuts alkaline mineral and soap deposits from surfaces. When the rinse water is used to water plants, it helps some water-soluble minerals in the soil dissolve and become available to plants.

Essential oils are added to the wash and rinse water for fragrance and anti-microbial properties. Any that remain in the water after cleaning may deter a few bugs that feed on plants when the gray water is carried out to the garden. This system of cleaning and plant care seems to be very agreeable to all concerned.

The essential oils are volatile and evaporate from dishes and other surfaces very quickly. Dishes, glasses, mugs and silverware washed and rinsed in this water do not retain the flavor of the oils or affect the taste of food or beverages.

We constantly vary essential oils in our **anti-microbial cleaning agent** and **anti-microbial vinegar** to confuse germs so that they do not build up immunity to our concoctions. Lemon oil smells "squeaky clean" to us. Orange oil is an emulsifier and is used in cleaning agents now available on the market. During flu season, we may use thyme or oregano oil to kill more germs. We think of the hot water as an essential oil steam diffuser. Peppermint oil stimulates the senses resulting in a peppy dishwashing experience. Conversely, lavender relaxes the mind and de-stresses the "washer." We make our formulas up as we go, depending upon the mood or motive of the moment when the bottles need refilling. This takes housecleaning to a whole new dimension.

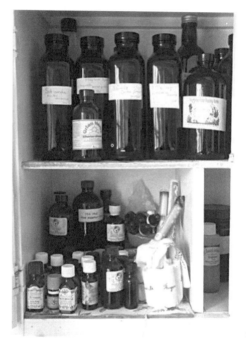

essential oils and household products made with them make housekeeping an aromatherapeutic experience

anti-microbial cleaning agent

We use this to wash dishes and other household surfaces. Re-used dishwashing detergent or gourmet vinegar bottles work nicely as dispensers because they have portion control tops. Though not necessary to make a good cleaning agent, the use of distilled water will result in less mineral sediment in the concoction.

3/4 cup distilled water
3/4 cup liquid surfactant or castile soap
10 drops essential oil, either oregano, peppermint, thyme or tea tree oil
5 drops lemon or orange essential oil for fragrance

Pour the water into the dispenser first to avoid foaming. Add surfactant or liquid castile soap. Add the essential oils. Put the lid on then turn the bottle upside down and back up several times to gently mix the ingredients before every use. Label the bottle.

Use about 1 tablespoon of cleaning agent in your dishwashing basin and fill with hot water.

Keep out of reach of children (until they are old enough to do chores.)

Tip: Susan mixes this up and lets her teenage daughters choose EOs that they like and they keep it by their bathroom sink for washing hands.

anti-microbial vinegar

It is best to store vinegar in glass with a plastic lid such as re-used, pint-size glass vinegar bottles. Vinegar corrodes metal lids and creates a deadly poison when left in contact with copper or lead.

2 cups apple cider vinegar
10 drops essential oil: choose either oregano, thyme, tea tree, rosemary, tangerine or lemon oil

Measure the essential oil drops into the vinegar. Label the bottle. *Keep out of reach of children.* Shake well before every use. Put about 1 to 2 tablespoons in your rinse water when rinsing dishes or kitchen and bath surfaces.

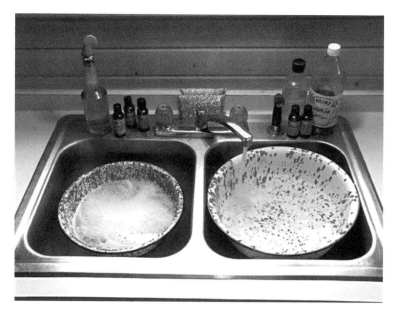

wash and rinse water for dishes using our anti-microbial cleaning agent & anti-microbial vinegar

washing vegetables

Before consuming fruits, vegetables and herbs it is necessary to wash them. Organisms that cause food-borne disease and disagreeable gritty soil must be removed before the food is fit to eat.

E. coli, the abbreviated name for *Escherichia coli* and specifically the problematic strain, 0157:H7 *E. coli* is a bacterium contracted from contaminated surfaces and food. It contains a virus in its DNA that produces a toxin in the intestines known as Vero toxin or Shiga-like toxin (SLT).

It weakens intestinal walls, causes cramping, diarrhea and hemorrhaging. The symptoms of infection usually show up within three to five days after the ingestion of the bacteria and include low-grade fever, vomiting, and in particular, the presence of blood in the stool. If these symptoms are displayed, a physician should be called immediately. The disease can resolve itself in about eight days in otherwise healthy adults, but infected persons can develop permanent kidney failure, especially children, the elderly and infirmed persons.

Scientist Susan Sumner, while working at the University of Nebraska, tested an effective method for killing harmful bacteria, including 0157:H7 *E. coli* on food. Apple cider or distilled white vinegar and 3 % hydrogen peroxide are the disinfectants. Use separate plastic spray bottles (available in the garden or cosmetic section of stores) for each liquid. Do not mix them together and do not dilute them with water. Label your sprayers. To wash vegetables and kitchen surfaces, simply spritz with both sprays; it doesn't matter in what order you spray them. Rinse with fresh water. Since hydrogen peroxide destroys microbes on contact, it is safe to use the rinse water on plants.

Another study of interest is the Japanese article published by Nakano Central Research Institute of Nakano Vinegar Co. Ltd. online at www.Pubmed.com. It reported that grain and rice vinegar, at 0.1% acidity inhibit the growth of bacteria but the 0157:H7 *E. coli* is resistive to acidity. Spirit (or pickling) vinegar at 10% acidity, and warmed to just over 100° Fahrenheit killed the greatest number of 0157:H7 *E. coli*. Most commercially available vinegar is has only 5% acidity but can be reduced down by boiling to half the volume, which doubles the acidity.

We remove dirt and bacteria from garden greens and pre-washed salad mixes by using vinegar and hydrogen peroxide in the wash water. Run water into the container bowl of a salad spinner. Add several tablespoons of vinegar. Place the greens in the spinner basket and immerse them in the acidified (vinegared) water. Gently agitate the greens for several minutes then lift the basket out of the water.

Repeat with fresh water and vinegar if needed, until the greens are free of grit. The acidulated water causes the grit to slip off of the greens and fall to the bottom of the bowl. Refill the container bowl with water, add several tablespoons of hydrogen peroxide and repeat the washing sequence as above. Finally, fill the bowl with fresh water, rinse the leaves and spin dry. All of the water used for washing and rinsing greens can be used to water plants.

household insect repellents

Living in homes cooled by shade trees and breezes that blow through screened windows, we enjoy studying the world of bugs in our environment. Each insect or mite has to make a living and each is prey for another bug or bird or reptile. Generally trusting in the balance of nature, we consider recluse and black widow spiders, gypsy moths, fleas, ticks and mosquitoes the only creatures dangerous enough to kill on sight. Otherwise, we like to peacefully co-exist, watching how natural communities interact—to a point. That point usually comes during the dog days of summer when we retreat indoors from the heat of the garden to find that pests have invaded our homes. This is a time to take back the house.

Pest-repellent herbs work best when they are replaced with fresh ones seasonally and when used in conjunction with proper cleaning and storage. Freshly dried bay leaves deter miller moths from grains especially well when the food is kept in airtight containers in the refrigerator or freezer.

Clean wool items stored in airtight cedar closets and chests are protected from moth damage with sachets of fresh dried lavender, southernwood and/or wormwood. Fresh cut tansy and southernwood placed across well-sealed thresholds with screened doors, windows washed with **insect-repellent glass cleaner,** and floors mopped with **insect-repellent floor wash** will help repel ants, fleas and flying insects. Herbs and essential oils, used with common sense and good housekeeping skills will protect you and the contents of your home.

book-bug repellent alcohol

Tina and Susan both live in homes without air-conditioning. Dust, book bugs, and mold are problems in their extensive libraries. To combat these problems, they researched essential oils that would help them take care of one of their largest investments, their books. Eucalyptus kills mold, mildew, and dust mites. Patchouli is a repellent for book bugs and we think it smells kind of hip. Either rubbing alcohol or vodka is used as the carrier because it evaporates quickly without damaging the books.

1/2 cup isopropyl or ethyl alcohol
5 drops each eucalyptus and patchouli oil

Combine all ingredients in a clean 4-ounce blue or brown glass spray bottle. Label the bottle.

Shake well before using. Do not saturate books or finished surfaces with the alcohol. Spray it on a cleaning cloth to remove dust and to apply repellent oils to surfaces.

Store this on the book shelf so that it is within easy reach when you are getting a book down to read; The alcohol will not go bad in storage but the essential oils may deteriorate in time.

Caution: Keep out of reach of children. Beware that some essential oils can damage plexiglass and varnished wood surfaces. Always test cleaning and insect-repellent agents on an inconspicuous area before applying to the entire surface. Alcohol can be irritating to mucous membranes and drying to the skin.

insect-repellent glass cleaner

Citrus oils have degreasing properties and they tend to make the window washer feel more cheerful. Vinegar is a traditional solvent for cleaning glass. Using this combination, grime and fly-specks are quickly cut away. We use glass spray bottles from used window-cleaner dispensers for our homemade glass cleaner. Clear plastics are broken down by essential oils. Choose thick-walled colored plastic for this purpose if glass cannot be found.

1 pint distilled white or apple cider vinegar
10 drops sweet orange oil

Measure the vinegar and essential oil into a clean spray bottle. Shake well before using. Label the bottle.

Spray the vinegar on the glass, working in quadrants from the top, working down. Polish the surface with a clean, lint-free cloth until it is dry and free of streaks.

Use this within one year for best results. The vinegar will not go bad; however, the essential oils may lose potency in storage. *Store with your other cleaning supplies; keep out of reach of children.*

Note: Any product that you make containing essential oils should be stored in a dark place, since light destroys EOs.

insect-repellent floor wash

Have an aromatherapeutic experience while scrubbing your floor; this one is head-clearing!

1 gallon warm water
1/4 cup surfactant, Murphy's Oil Soap®, Dr. Bronner's Sal Suds or castile soap
10 drops each orange and eucalyptus oil
1 drop vetiver oil

Pour warm water into a bucket. Add the rest of the ingredients and mix well. Vacuum floor surfaces before washing or mopping and discard refuse in a sealed trash bag. Wearing rubber gloves, clean the floor and allow to air dry.

Note: Keep your pets free of fleas and ticks. If you are fighting fleas, repeat vacuuming and mopping every 3 days to destroy adult fleas as their eggs, larvae and pupae mature.

Tip: Mature fleas are attracted to light. To trap and kill them, place a shallow pan of soapy water on the floor in the infested area. Place a lamp or secure a low-voltage light bulb above the pan of water. The fleas will hop in and drown. This is a good way to eliminate breeding fleas and monitor the success of your flea control methods. *Caution: To avoid any electrical accidents, make certain that the light source is secure and cannot fall into the water.*

moth-repellent alcohol

We use this fast-drying repellent on wool socks, blankets and sweaters. Before summer storage, the articles are first washed in cold water with a non-alkaline detergent such as Woolite® or a surfactant such as Shaklee's Basic H®. We spray the damp woolens lightly with the repellent and then lay them flat to dry. Woolens are stored in airtight trunks or cedar chests until needed again.

1/2 cup isopropyl or ethyl alcohol
10 drops lavender oil
1 drop vetiver oil

Combine all ingredients in a clean 4-ounce blue or brown glass spray bottle. Shake well before using. Lightly spray this on the wool when it is damp or dry. Store the repellent in a cool, dark place for up to one year. Label the bottle. *Caution: Keep out of reach of children.*

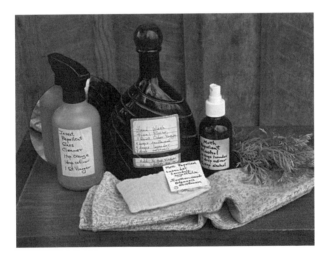

household preparations: insect-repellent glass cleaner, anti-microbial vinegar, & moth-repellent alcohol

all-purpose bathroom scrub

This isn't really a set recipe, since it just requires baking soda and a few drops of essential oil. Baking soda is abrasive and not harmful to our environment as are harsh scouring powders with bleach. For scouring sinks, tubs, shower stalls and toilets—just sprinkle in the baking soda, shake in a few drops of tea tree for disinfectant purposes, perhaps lemon, orange or grapefruit for that clean citrus aroma—and use a sponge, scrubby or toilet brush to remove grime and/or soap or oil scum. Rinse well with warm water.

(For a science project experiment, we like to spray the baking soda with vinegar and watch the alkaline and acid neutralize one another.)

Tip: Where Susan lives in Maryland, she gets heavy blue mineral deposits on her bathroom fixtures. She has tried many products trying to remove the blue stains. Recently her niece Sara reported that she had found a natural way to get rid of these deposits. Sara often uses our bath salts in her tub and she found that after soaking in the tub with our **well body bath salts** *made from Epsom salts with EOs of rosemary, eucalyptus, and peppermint, not only did she feel great, but her tub was totally free of mineral stains!*

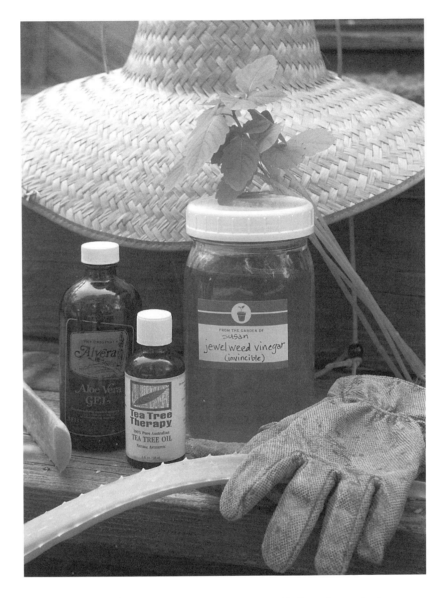

*gardening comforts: aloe vera, tea tree oil, jewelweed vinegar —
and of course, straw hat and gardening gloves*

gardening comforts

With the joy of gardening and all other outdoor summer recreation comes the challenge of staying comfortable—and protecting ourselves from biting bugs, harmful sunrays, and irritating plant oils—and healing the damage that is done to our largest organ, the skin. To be at ease in the great out-of-doors, we have to be smarter and more disciplined than the natural forces in and around us. Physical discomforts contracted from nature can be modified but never entirely conquered. We can reduce contact with the pests and speed the healing of the hurts to reduce suffering.

Our first line of defense is internal. We eat lots of garlic. We increase our intake of vitamin C during the gardening season for energy and a healthy immune system and we drink large amounts of water. If we get the beginning of a poison ivy/oak rash, or incur bug bites, we use echinacea tincture for several days to boost our immune systems.

There are plentiful pests to humans in the garden: mosquitoes, "no-see-'ems" (biting gnats), biting flies, chiggers and ticks, to name a few. There are allergic reactions to poison ivy, rue, okra and squash leaves and other individual allergies. Sun and heat, wind, as well as perpetually wet feet are all challenges to a happy, productive attitude. Before we step out of the door we dress, from the skin out, in a manner appropriate to the outside conditions and the planned activities of the day.

Tina Marie, who is a dedicated, full-time gardener at the Ozark Folk Center, in Mountain View, Arkansas uses physical barriers against sun, bugs and poison ivy/oak and other plants that contain furocoumarins (see **plant chemicals**) oils as she works in her Ozark gardens. Before she gets dressed, she applies **antiseptic insect repellent oil** to her entire body. She wears white, long-sleeved cotton blouses and trousers, gloves, and boots. She tucks her trousers into the tops of her boots and secures the cuffs to her ankles with elastic straps that fasten with Velcro™. (These are available in the sporting goods section of stores.) Tina Marie waterproofs her leather boots and gloves with **insect repellent neatsfoot oil**. She dusts her feet and the inside of her boots with **gardener's foot powder** to deter bugs, athletes' foot fungus, and absorb perspiration. White cotton tea towels, sprayed with **insect repellent vinegar** and draped around her neck absorb perspiration and reflect sunrays. Finally, she tops off her gardening uniform with a wide-brimmed straw hat.

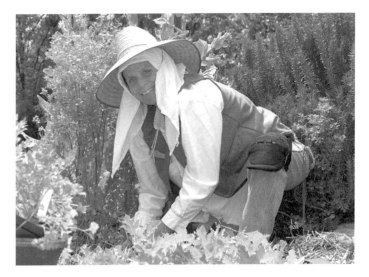

Tina Marie in her gardener's garb

On the other hand, Susan is more of a casual gardener, who is most comfortable wearing minimal clothing and going barefoot in the garden. Because of this practice, she takes a lot of outdoor showers, uses sunblock protection and does wear a hat in the middle of the day. She tends to work outside in the morning and evening rather than the heat of the day, when possible. She regularly uses **jewelweed vinegar with insect repellent herbs** before heading out to the garden, which keeps the biting flies and mosquitoes away. Of course, for tough chores and going into the woods, she suits up as described above as any sensible girl would.

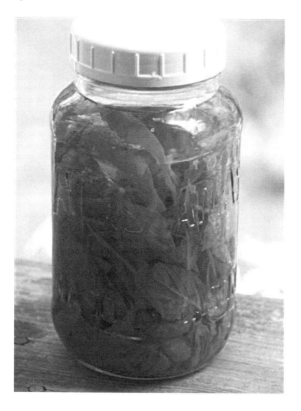

jewelweed vinegar (otherwise known as invincible vinegar)

sunburn

Protecting our skin against the sun is very important. In the summer, we like to wear less clothing and feel the summer sun or the sea breeze on our bare skin. If we do so, we really need to use some kind of sunblock.

After a day outside in the sun—even if we use sunblock—but especially if you don't, the result can be sunburn. There are a number of remedies to cool sunburn and *Aloe vera* is one of our favorites. You can cut a leaf from your aloe plant, slit it open and use the sap directly on the skin, or scrape it from the leaf and mix it with a little water and vitamin E oil for easier application and to make it go a little farther. A bottle of aloe vera gel, available at the health food store, works too; keep either in the refrigerator— wrap the leaf so it doesn't dry out. We also use it for small first and second-degree burns, often adding a drop or two of organic lavender oil. All-purpose herbal salve or jewelweed vinegar diluted with three parts water can also be used on sunburn.

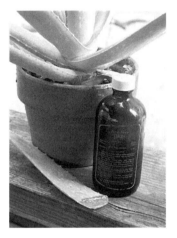

aloe vera plant or gel cools sunburn and kitchen burns

speeding the healing

When insects bite, athlete's foot fungus is among us or toxic plant oils get under our skin, we make it our mission to heal as quickly as possible. The worst thing to do is to give in to the itch caused by histamines and scratch. Scratching inflames the wound, causes more itching and prolongs the healing process by introducing secondary infections. We use a battery of remedies to shorten the duration of the torment and to keep an alternative to scratching close at hand.

Tea tree oil, distilled from the Australian tree, *Melaleuca alternifolia*, is with us at all times, especially during chigger and tick season. We rub a bit of the oil on the bites when they itch because we both know from experience that we can apply it neat to our skin.

Applying herbal salves, tinctures or tea tree oil answers the itchy demand for attention with out scratching. *Caution: Do not use an oil-based salve on an open wound. Do a* **patch test** *(see* **definition of terms**) *before applying tea tree oil directly on your skin.*

Caution: Always test for individual allergic reactions to homemade substances before applying them to large areas of the body. A **simple skin test** *is to drop a little of the concoction on the inner arm (elbow crease is convenient) and wait 30 minutes to an hour, especially if you have allergies or sensitive skin. If the skin does not redden or blister, you should be good to go.*

chiggers, mosquitoes and ticks

Chiggers, also known as red bugs, *Thrombicula alfredduges* are soft-bodied mites that pester gardeners in the eastern United States. They perch on the tops of plants and wait for prey. As we work in the garden, chiggers climb onto our bodies, find a nice tender place and insert their mouthparts into the skin. It is a myth that they burrow in and live under the skin. The chigger larval stage feeds by injecting an enzyme into the epidermis. The enzyme simultaneously breaks down the skin cells and creates intense itching at the site of the bite. The foremost thing to bear in mind is that the mite has a soft body. To kill many of them before they bite you, simply hand-rub your skin and clothes often by brushing up and down, when working in the garden.

Mosquitoes and ticks inflict itchy bites that can become infected, but even worse, they and carry seriously debilitating diseases. Mosquitoes are most active at dawn and dusk and in shady, moist areas. They need standing water to reproduce. To control their numbers, eliminate standing water as much as possible, and consider using "Bt" (*Bacillius thuringiensis* var. *israelensis*,) a bacterial larvicide applied to ponds, rain barrels and bird feeders. Bt is harmless to all life forms except the larvae of mosquitoes, fungus gnats and black flies.

Though ticks are active through the mild days of winter, they tend to be most active in the heat of summer where animals such as deer, cattle and even lizards roam, serving as hosts for feeding and breeding. Adjust the timing and location of your gardening activities to keep yourself safe from harm. Use wide masking tape to stick and capture ticks that walk on you.

Remember to combine frequent 'tick checks' and chigger killing with water breaks. Be familiar with the symptoms associated with tick and mosquito-born diseases. When you do get bites, treat them aggressively and seek prompt medical attention if disease symptoms occur.

We shower as often as possible during the day to rinse biting bugs from our bodies. We apply **antiseptic insect-repellent skin oil** several times a day. The essential oils speed the healing of bites and repel insects as they volatilize. The carrier oil smothers pests by shutting off their breathing apparatus in the exoskeleton of their bodies. We think that if biting bugs light on oiled skin they don't like that oily feeling on their little feet and proboscis. The moisturizing and therapeutic effects of the oil are enjoyable as it protects us from some insect bites. This protection may last an hour.

there ain't no bugs on me

The insect-repellent essential oils we find are most cost effective and useful are citronella, eucalyptus, lavender and Texas cedarwood. Rose geranium, lemongrass, patchouli, sandalwood and vetiver are also effective against bugs in our environment. These oils, diluted in a carrier such as skin-nourishing seed oils, vinegar or witch hazel seem to be effective against mosquitoes, gnats, chiggers, ticks and biting flies. We have not found a repellent that is 100% effective. Essential oils are volatile by nature; this means they evaporate quickly and must be reapplied regularly to work.

antiseptic insect-repellent skin oil

Avoid applying this preparation to mucus membranes, your eyes, open wounds and rashes. Oregano, thyme and tea tree are very strong and pungent essential oils, so we suggest a skin test first; if it burns when you apply it, do not use it or dilute it with more carrier oil.

1/2 cup almond, walnut or grape seed oil
5 drops oregano, thyme or tea tree oil
5 drops rose geranium, lavender, lemon balm, peppermint or lemon grass oil

Pour the carrier oil into a clean, dark glass bottle and then drop in a total of 10 drops of essential oils. Tighten the lid and shake well before every use. Label bottle. *Keep out of reach of children.*

Tina uses this oil all over her body before dressing for garden work. Reapply to exposed skin when insects bite. Keep the bottle in a cool place and use it within two weeks.

Caution: Always test products containing essential oils on the inside of the arm before applying to larger areas of the body. (see **skin test** in **definition of terms**)

Be not afraid: By using common sense, discipline and our green friends, the herbs, we can work and play outdoors with confidence and relative comfort.

insect repellent herbal vinegar

We pour our vinegars into spray bottles for easy application.

2 cups fresh insect repellent herbs
2 cups apple cider vinegar

Crush the herbs with a mortar and pestle. Place herbs in a clean, glass quart jar and cover with vinegar. Use a plastic lid to seal the jar (vinegar corrodes metal). Shake everyday for 3 to 7 days. It is best to filter the vinegar in a week and use it up within the year.

The essential oils of the plants are volatile and degrade with time. Store the vinegar in a cool, dark place. Label bottle. *Keep out of reach of children.*

The following herbs are some of our favorite insect repellents:

catnip (*Nepeta cataria*)
East Indian lemongrass (*Cymbopogon flexuosus*)
eucalyptus (*Eucalyptus globulus*)
lemon balm (*Melissa officinalis*)
lemon eucalyptus (*Eucalyptus citriodora*)
lavender (*Lavandula angustifolia* and *L.* x *intermedia*)
lemon thyme (*Thymus* x*citriodorus*)
mountain mint (*Pycnanthemum albescens*)

Note: In a study from the University of Iowa, researchers found that the chemical nepetalactone found in catnip is 10 times more effective than Deet at repelling mosquitoes. So try some in your insect-repellent vinegar, or try rubbing some catnip on exposed areas before going outside.

the creative herbal home

feet first

insect-repellent neat's-foot oil

To discourage biting bugs from hitching a ride, we waterproof our leather boots with this combination. It can also use it on leather gardening gloves and leather tool pouches.

1/2 teaspoon each eucalyptus and citronella essential oils
7 1/2 fluid ounces bottle neat's-foot oil

Measure the EOs directly into the neat's-foot oil bottle and shake well before each use. Apply to clean leather boots with a cloth. The leather will darken. Do not use on suede leather. Store in a cool dark place. The storage life of this repellent is indefinite; however, it will repel more bugs when applied to boots rather than left to sit in the bottle. Tip: Keep the application cloth in a labeled, sealed container so it can be used again. Label bottle. *Keep out of reach of children.*

gardener's foot powder

Athlete's foot fungus loves damp conditions caused by perspiration and watering chores. Lavender and tea tree combat the fungus and the powders absorb moisture.

1/4 cup cornstarch
1/4 cup baking soda
10 drops each lavender and tea tree oil
Measure all ingredients into a small bowl. Mix thoroughly and store in an airtight container. Dust feet lightly before putting on shoes and after bathing. Store in a cool, dark place. Use within one year. Label jar. *Keep out of reach of children.*

peacefully coexisting with poison ivy and poison oak

First, learn the rule, "leaves of three, let it be" to identify poison ivy and poison oak. It is faster to walk around it than it is to heal the rash. Wear gloves in the garden as much as possible and don boots and long pants before going into the woods. If you discover you have been walking or working in poison ivy (*Toxicodendron radicans* and *T. rydbergii*) or poison oak (*T. toxicarium* and *T. diversilobum*), it is important to remove the oil from the skin as soon as possible. Susan washes with *Fels Naptha®* (yellow soap) that is kept by the laundry sink in her mudroom and by her outdoor shower, as soon as she gets back to the house. She rinses all the way up her arms and down again with cold water. If she has been wearing flip-flops or barefoot, then she scrubs up to her knees and back down. If she thinks she may have touched her face or neck, she washes them too. It is important to pat dry, don't rub. Wash tools, gloves, shoes and all clothing, and then, wash your hands again.

Next, she immediately uses one of the following to break the oil (urishiol) on the skin if there is any remaining: alcohol, jewelweed vinegar or witch hazel. Splash them all over liberally. We've tried using all of them and this extra step really does seem to help prevent getting the rash. Our favorite is jewelweed vinegar, however it does have the strongest odor. We believe it really works.

If you develop poison ivy rash, take these steps to heal quickly. Dry the blisters, sooth the inflammation and kill microbes that cause secondary infections. Drying agents include alcohol, witch hazel, vinegar, oatmeal and green clay. The very best remedy for drying up poison ivy is going to the beach and swimming in the salty ocean; it really does wonders. Alternatively, take a tepid shower or soak in a bath with oatmeal or baking soda added. After patting dry, we apply jewelweed vinegar, or anti-microbial washes such as alcohol or witch hazel, and antiseptic and anti-inflammatory herbal infusions. When we are in the throes of blistering, we add herbal infusions to oatmeal or green clay to make a paste and slather this on the rash. Both of these are very drying — once dried, rinse off, and *rub gently* to remove residue.

Our water or vinegar infusions are made with mucilage-containing, anti-inflammatory and astringent herbs such as calendula, jewelweed, comfrey, flax seed, aloe vera, oatmeal, mullein, yarrow and plantain. These sooth the rash and leave a protective barrier on the skin when they dry.

We add antiseptic herbs and essential oils to boost the germ-killing properties of our infusions. We think about what we have on hand, study our herbals and make the remedies to maintain the focus on healing rather than scratching.

When the rash dries up, the second phase of ivy treatment is to use salves and creams to help the tissues heal. *Oil-based remedies trap moisture in the skin and are best used after the blisters have dried up, so do not use them on open sores or scabs.*

jewelweed vinegar

Jewelweed, *Impatiens capensis*, is a native plant in the eastern United States that grows mostly in wet places. The plant's juice is a handy remedy for any itchy skin irritation. It grows in our gardens during the summer. We simply crush the stems and leaves, then apply the juice to rashes and bites. Preserve the plant's juice in vinegar to keep it handy for use at any time. Vinegar is antibacterial and stings a bit. We use organic apple cider vinegar when we prepare this and refer to this infusion as *invincible vinegar*.

2 cups apple cider vinegar
1 cup fresh crushed jewelweed

Place the jewelweed in a clean, glass quart jar. Cover with vinegar and seal the jar with a plastic lid (vinegar corrodes metal). Label the jar; *keep out of reach of children*. Shake everyday for 3 days.

Strain the vinegar through cheesecloth. Store jewelweed vinegar in a tightly sealed, dark-glass container. As we need it, we pour the vinegar into a spray bottle for easy application. Vinegar will attract vinegar flies if left unsealed. After one year the jewelweed vinegar seems to lose some potency. Make fresh every season.

Variation: After straining, add ten drops each insect repellent and antiseptic essential oils to one-pint of the vinegar. We pour the vinegar into a spray bottle for easy application. We use the spray to treat itchy skin conditions and to revitalize the repellent "cloud" around us.

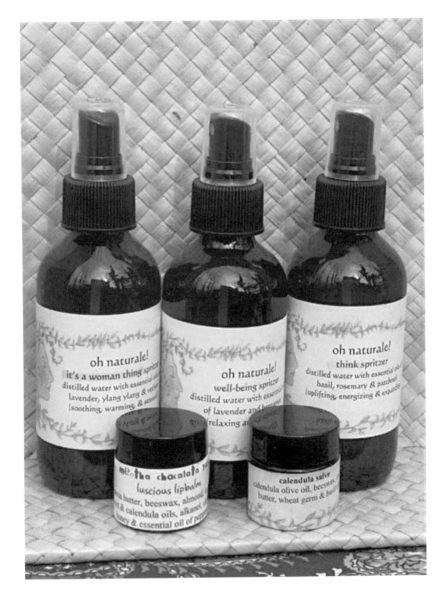

*homemade body care products: aromatherapy spritzers,
mentha chocolata lip balm, and herbal salve*

body care

The ingredients for making body care products should be of a very high quality from our own organically grown gardens or vendors that support our vision for the world. All are simply from the earth and her plants. We will make these products from our own imagination—intimate knowledge of our friends and family members—with our own hands. The packaging should be appropriate to the created product.

spritzers

Our spritzers are elegantly simple—made with distilled water and aromatic essential oils—and intent to support positive thinking, empowering the user to alter environmental and emotional circumstances by briefly changing the molecules in the air. (More study in the therapeutic benefits of essential oils is recommended: see **sources**.) We mail order 4-ounce blue glass bottles with spray nozzles. Susan designs the labels for her spritzers under the business name *oh naturale!* and prints them from her computer. Tina buys large gold stick-on stars from office supply stores and hand writes her labels.

Since spritzers are made with distilled water and aromatic essential oils, they are not strong and long lasting like perfume. Once spritzed, they aromatherapize the air and then dissipate quickly. Since oil and water do not mix, the essential oil drops float on top of the distilled water, therefore, the spritzers need to be shaken before using. We use our spritzers often, so they do not set too long. If you are keeping spritzers for more than a month or so, there is a chance for bacteria or mold to grow, even though the water is distilled. One teaspoon of alcohol added to each spritzer bottle will help to inhibit the growth of bacteria, although it will alter the fragrance of the spritzer. Spritzers will keep longer in the fridge—which is nice in the summertime.

Spritzers, sometimes referred to as mists, are designed to lift our spirits and give pleasure, whether you need soothing, uplifting or stimulating. Spritz your body, clothes or the air around you. Once spritzed, the EOs dissipate rather quickly. Lavender has anti-bacterial, antibiotic, antiseptic, and anti-viral attributes, so it helps guard against germs of all kinds, which make these spritzers great for using around the house, office, cars, airplanes and hotel rooms.

When creating spritzers or any body care products, look for EOs that work for your specific need or choose ones that you like. We often test fragrance combinations with perfumer's test strips or by holding the EO bottles we are combining and take a gentle whiff to see how they work together. If you aren't happy with the combination, take one EO away, and try another in its place.

When creating a harmonizing blend think about balancing the aromas so that they work together and compliment one another. For instance, in **the it's a woman thing spritzer** blend, the middle note is lavender and there are 7 drops. Ylang-ylang is very exotic, feminine and floral, so we use just 3 drops. To balance the flowery top note of ylang-ylang, we need an earthy note. Vetiver is very earthy, musk-like, and powerful. We use just one drop so as not to overpower the other EOs. It's fun and enjoyable to create your own blends. Two or three, at most four, essential oils are good to start. When you use too many EOs your fragrance can become overwhelming or muddy.

Susan created the following blends to suit the described needs. They are some of her favorite synergistic blends.

basic spritzer instructions

When preparing any of the spritzers below, drop your EOs into a 4-ounce spritzer bottle first, then carefully pour the water in. Cap, shake and spritz. Adjust with a few more drops of EO if necessary and label. Use within a month or two; shake well before using. *Keep out of reach of children.*

soothing spritzer (relaxing and calming)

4 ounces distilled water
About 6 drops lavender essential oil
3 to 4 drops rose or rose geranium essential oil

When we need to soothe others or ourselves we use this spritzer—it balances and calms—we spritz when our nerves are tense. We use this spritz if we're feeling sad, mad, hurt, anxious or emotional. It is great before presentations, on airplanes and in traffic jams. Susan often spritzes her teenagers' rooms with this, especially when emotions or tempers are out of balance.

well-being spritzer (relaxing and uplifting)

4 ounces distilled water
About 6 drops lavender essential oil
About 7 drops bergamot essential oil

We spritz with this when we need a pick-me-up—at mid-morning or afternoon slump—or after lunch. It promotes a general well being of spirit, so we use it around the house, in the office, or before and after doing errands.

stimulating spritzer (relaxing and head-clearing)

4 ounces distilled water
About 6 drops lavender essential oil
About 7 drops rosemary essential oil

When we need to change our state of mind or concentrate, we spritz with this—before or during a brainstorming session—around the kids at homework time. We use it to clear out the cobwebs, when feeling like a nap and still have to things to accomplish. We also spray this in the bathrooms and kids' rooms during the cold and flu season, and after a germ-infested guest comes to visit.

it's a woman thing spritzer (relaxing and balancing)

4 ounces distilled water
About 7 drops lavender essential oil
About 3 drops ylang ylang essential oil
About 1 drop vetiver essential oil

We often spritz with this before going downstairs in the morning— before leaving the house—and before the kids come home from school. We use it when feeling indecisive, when nerves are frazzled or when feeling emotional or out-of-sorts. Good for PMS, pre- and post- menopausal symptoms.

think spritzer (uplifting, energizing, and expanding)

4 ounces distilled water
About 6 drops basil essential oil
About 6 drops rosemary essential oil
About 1 drop patchouli essential oil

This is a blend that Tina Marie came up with; it is good when we really have to think or concentrate and get a job done. If we're tired, stressed out or feeling indecisive or nervous, it helps us to put things into perspective, feel confident, and balance body and mind. We find it helps when we need a real lift or pick-me-up and need to get going! This is a sit-up and take-notice kind of spritz.

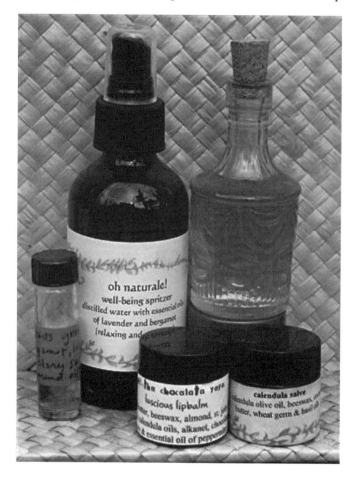

aromatherapy spritzer and herbal spa products

mentha chocolata yaya luscious lip balm

When Susan did her herbal apprenticeship with Rosemary Gladstar, the class was divided into groups to make salves, oils and balms for different maladies. The assignment was to formulate an herbal product to treat a specific problem, design a label for it and make an advertisement. Susan's group was assigned a lip balm— they had to make a batch of 40 so that everyone could have one.

The fragrance of the cocoa butter inspired the use of the organic chocolate bar; Susan just happened to have a Dagoba bar with her. As the fun progressed, so did the creativity and they formed the "Herbal Yaya Sisters." They sang their advertisement to the tune of Patti Labelle's Lady Marmalade—you know the one *"Mocha Chocolata Yaya"*—with quite a bit of lip puckering.

Here is the ad that the Herbal Yayas wrote about their product:
Mentha Chocolata Yaya Lip Balm
"The quintessential balm for the most luscious of lips!
~ You will love this sensuous, lip-smacking combination of bittersweet chocolate with just a hint of peppermint.
~ The Herbal Yayas use only the finest ingredients—almond oil and cocoa butter to seal and protect lips—and lend a yummy fragrance and flavor.
~ *Alkanet* adds emollient and sunscreen properties and just the sheerest tint for ruby red lips.
~ *Saint-John's-wort oil* is added for a sunscreen. *Caution: In our original recipe we used Saint-John's-wort oil. However, in researching this book we found the following quote by Foster and Duke in Eastern Medicinal Plants: "taken internally or externally, hypericin may cause phytodermatitis (skin burns) in sensitive persons exposed to sunlight." So we recommend using olive, grape seed or almond oil in its place to be safe.*

~ *Calendula oil* has wonderful healing and soothing properties.
~ *Organic bittersweet chocolate* is a food of the gods and of course, tastes good too.
~ *Essential oil of peppermint* is uplifting and stimulating—not that you'll need any stimulation—because your lips will be so kissable they will be getting lots of action"!

Prepared in small batches and made from the finest ingredients, the following recipe can be halved to make a smaller amount. The recipe for herbal oil is below.

Makes enough to fill about 45 .15-ounce standard lip balm tubes or 24 1/4-ounce pots

1/2 cup almond oil
1 tablespoon olive oil, grape seed or St.-John's-wort oil
3 tablespoons calendula oil
1/2 cup cocoa butter
1 ounce organic bittersweet chocolate (about 57 to 60% cocoa), cut into bits
1 teaspoon honey
1/4 cup alkanet
1/4 cup natural beeswax pellets, or grated beeswax
8 drops essential oil of peppermint

In the top of a double boiler over simmering water, combine the almond, olive oil or St.-John's-wort and calendula oils with the cocoa butter, chocolate, honey and alkanet. Stir until the cocoa butter and chocolate have melted; reduce heat and let stand for about 30 minutes so that the color of the alkanet is extracted. Be sure that the water doesn't bubble away in the bottom of the double boiler.

Pour the contents of the double boiler through a strainer lined with a double layer of dampened cheesecloth into a bowl. Press on or squeeze the excess liquid from the cheesecloth—be careful, as alkanet is a red dye that stains even countertops. Return the strained oil mixture to the double boiler and add the beeswax, and increase the heat to medium to melt the beeswax. *(Do not miss this step: If you add the beeswax—and then try to strain out the alkanet—it will be too thick.)*

Once the beeswax is melted, do a test for consistency by putting just a bit on a spoon or a saucer and placing it in the fridge. It should harden in about 2, at most 5, minutes. You don't want it to be too hard, but it shouldn't be liquid. If you feel it is too thin, you can add a little more beeswax. Once you are satisfied with the consistency, remove the pan from the heat and stir in the peppermint oil. Pour while hot into small pots or carefully into lip balm tubes. Let stand without lids until cool, then cap, label and store away from heat. Use within 3 months; store extras in fridge for longer shelf life.

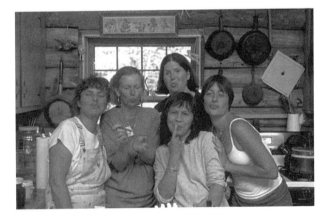

herbal yayas: Susan Belsinger, Debby Jennings, Shakti Colin, Linda Russell, & Kim Xenakis

calendula oil

One oil that we prepare every summer is calendula oil. Calendula is a wonderful herb for the skin. We harvest calendula petals as they peak and dry them over about a 4- to 6-week period. Herb-infused oils are easier to prepare with freshly dried herbs rather than fresh herbs, since there is less chance of fermentation due to water content in fresh material. The oil is a pretty yellow color and smells like the height of summer.

We use it all year long on our skin after we have showered applying when the skin is still moist, in massage oils and herbal salves, on boo-boos and bruises, and chapped lips. We prepare other herbal oils, like St.-John's-wort using the flowers and arnica using the leaves, following this recipe.

Measure chopped, dried calendula petals into a clean glass jar; the ratio is about 1 part herb to 4 parts oil.

Pour the oil (we use olive or almond oil) over the herbs, covering them completely. Place the jar(s) into a yogurt maker or turkey roaster (the temperature needs to remain between 110 and 120° F) and leave them for 10 days to 2 weeks, stirring everyday. The oil will become infused with the aroma and color of the herb.

Strain the finished oil through cheesecloth into a clean jar pressing on the herb to remove the essence. If there is any extra particulate in the oil, let it sit overnight and pour off the clear oil, leaving anything that settled in the bottom behind.

Label the oil, and store in a cool dark place for up to 1 year.

some herbs and essential oils for dry skin

These will vary according to each individual and their skin type: aloe vera, calendula, comfrey, chamomile, coltsfoot, dandelion, elder flowers, fennel, geranium, lavender, red clover, rose, sandalwood, ylang-ylang.

Xerosis is the medical term for dry skin, which is due to a lack of moisture in the skin. This occurs most often in the winter months when the humidity is low, and the outside air is cold while the inside is heated, as well as living in dry climates. Most often, it affects our arms and hands, lower and upper legs, feet, and sometimes the torso. Symptoms may include itching, cracks in the skin, and sometimes scaling. Generally, dry skin is not a serious condition; however, if it seems excessive, contact your health care provider because it may be something more serious.

Basically, moisturizer or cream holds water in the skin and acts as a barrier. Creams and lotions need to have water as an ingredient in order to hydrate the skin. Water hydrates; oils are not hydrating, but they soothe, seal and protect the skin. Read labels on your moisturizer.

Oil-in-water types contain more water and don't feel as greasy. These are good for sensitive skin types, like teenagers and young adults, or those who have a tendency to break out. Water-in-oil moisturizers should be used for dry skin and more mature skin, since they are richer and more lubricating, more like a face cream.

Some things that cause dry skin are: Lack of water; central heating, space heaters, woodstoves, even air-conditioning; weather like exposure to wind, cold, and sun; poor diet; sometimes a lack of omega-3s, vitamin A, and possibly zinc; alcohol, caffeine, and some prescription drugs such as antihistamines and diuretics.

Long, hot showers and baths dry out your skin by breaking down the lipid barriers, as does swimming in chlorinated pools; harsh soaps, detergents, and chemicals take both water and lipids from the skin. Antibacterial and deodorant soaps can be the most harmful; products with preservatives, fragrance, and lauryl sulfates tend to irritate and dry the skin more.

Ways to avoid dry skin are: Hydrate, drink water throughout the day; think about using a humidifier, if the air is dry in your home, it will dry out your skin; moisturize your home, for instance keep a large pot of water on the woodstove whenever it is going; lessen time spent in the shower and bath—use warm water, rather than hot—bathe less frequently; use less soap and limit it to hands and feet, underarms, genitals, and face. Non-detergent products with a neutral pH are better for the skin. Once out of the tub or shower, gently pat dry; do not rub or scrub your skin. Follow immediately with moisturizer or lotion while the skin is still damp, which will help capture and hold water in the surface cells of the skin.

Wear natural fabrics to allow your skin to breathe. Although wool is natural, it can be quite scratchy and irritating to some skin, so wear it as an outer layer, not up against the skin. Use fragrance and dye-free laundry detergent; always use sunscreen when out in the sun. A good well-balanced diet and exercise will benefit the skin. Exercise helps blood flow and circulation and helps to nourish and clean the skin.

homemade moisturizing cream

This recipe is adapted from *Rosemary Gladstar's FAMILY HERBAL*, which is a wonderful, must-have resource book. She calls it 'Rosemary's Perfect Cream' and it is quite rich and emollient. You can use any single oil or combination of oils and any combination of essential oils that are pleasing to you. It is best to make this cream in small quantities because when combining oil with water (even distilled water) there is the risk of microbes (bacteria/fungus) growing. In order to maintain freshness, store in a cool place or the refrigerator—and use within a month, two at the most—or add an anti-microbial preservative for a longer shelf life. For more information on preservatives, and a great source for ingredients, check out www.theherbarie.com.

Makes about 12-ounces of cream

1/4 cup almond oil
1/4 cup grape seed oil
1/4 cup cocoa butter
1/4 cup coarse-grated natural beeswax, tight-packed (about 3/4 ounce)
1/2 teaspoon vitamin E oil, optional
2/3 cup distilled water
1/4 cup aloe vera gel
6 to 10 drops essential oil (try 5 lavender, 3 sandalwood & 2 ylang-ylang, or create your own blend)

In the top of a double boiler, combine the almond and grape seed oils, cocoa butter, and beeswax. Place over medium heat and heat through until the cocoa butter and beeswax have just melted.

Remove the top of the double boiler from the bottom, stir in the vitamin E if you are using it, and set aside to cool. Combine the distilled water and aloe in a measuring cup; they should be at room temperature.

Once the oil mixture is almost cooled to room temperature, it will begin to thicken and almost solidify. Transfer the mixture to a clean blender and use a rubber scraper to scrape all of the oil mixture into the blender.

Both the oil mixture and the water mixture should be at room temperature before proceeding with the next step. Remember that oil and water don't mix, but we are going to make it happen. Turn the blender on and pour the water mixture into the center of movement in the blender. The mixture will be very thick, so you will have to stop the blender, scrape down the sides and stir the ingredients a few times. Add the essential oils during this process. If there is some water left standing on the emulsion, use the rubber scraper to fold it in.

Transfer the cream into a 12-ounce jar or two 6-ounce jars with lids that are scrupulously clean and label them. Store them in a cool place or refrigerate and use within 4 to 6 weeks.

If for some reason, your cream does not emulsify and separates, the oil and water mixtures were most likely not at room temperature. You can separate them and try to emulsify them again, or use as is, shaking before each use.

herb-scented lotion

Sometimes we add essential oils to good quality, fragrance-free lotion (that we purchase at our local health food stores, or from a favorite online herb source) to create a personal scent. You can make a variety of blends for different moods or design them for friends.

1 tablespoon almond oil or prepared calendula oil (see recipe above)
About 6 to 8 drops of essential oil
1/2 cup fragrance-free lotion

Put the almond oil in a small bowl. Drop the essential oil into the oil and stir well. Add the lotion and blend well. Transfer the lotion to a clean 4-ounce jar or bottle, place a lid on it and label. If there are no preservatives in this lotion, add one or use within a month or two; store in a cool place.

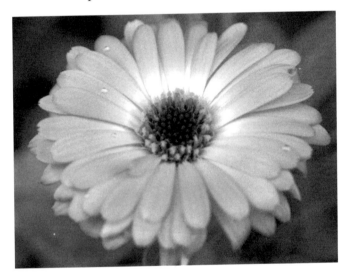

calendula flowers are a favorite herb for the skin

herbal bath therapy

An aromatic bath is one of the simplest and most pleasurable forms of herb therapy. Use fresh herbs and flowers, dried herbs and essential oils in the tub to create fragrant water therapy magic. Susan takes baths often—not because she is dirty—but because she enjoys the ritual. She feels that there is nothing more relaxing than a good hot soak in a scented tub.

bath oils and massage oils

We generally use almond or sesame oil and buy it in small amounts so it is fresh. Usually we blend two or three, sometimes four, different EOs together when making oil blends for the bath or massage. We use from 20 to 24 drops of essential oil to 2 ounces (about 4 tablespoons or 1/4 cup) of carrier oil, depending upon what we are doing with the oil. You can use more essential oil in a bath oil since it will be extremely diluted in a tub full of hot water. We use bath oils for cold symptoms (this works well on kids), muscle aches, to soothe and relax, to renew or to stimulate. A blend that we use for colds and flu is eucalyptus and lavender, with a drop or two of tea tree, and then one drop of peppermint or citrus EO. To relax in the tub, we use lavender, a little chamomile or ylang-ylang and just a drop or two of cedar or sandalwood.

For massage oil, we use much less essential oil because we don't want to overwhelm the person being massaged. Start with 6 to 10 drops to 2 ounces of oil, cap it and shake it up, and then rub a tiny bit on the back of your hand and sniff to see whether or not you want to add more essential oil. The act of massage is relaxing, and you can use oils to soothe, but you can also make blends that are warming or sensual. A very pleasant blend is lavender, sandalwood and just one drop of patchouli. We also like ylang-ylang or jasmine, which are fragrant and sensual with a little clary sage or cedarwood for balance.

marion's therapeutic massage oil

This recipe was passed on to us by our multi-talented friend Marion Spear and it is really deeply therapeutic. All of these essential oils are warming and will cause a hot sensation on the skin. It can be diluted with a bit more carrier oil if it is too strong— this is fairly intense and warming.

If you are new to using EOs, try it on a small spot of skin in your elbow crease and leave it there for 30 to 60 minutes; if it feels too hot then dilute it.

2 tablespoons (1 ounce) sweet almond or other fixed oil
10 drops ginger
10 drops rosemary
5 drops black pepper oil
5 drops peppermint

Put the almond oil in a small bottle and drop in the essential oils. Put the cap on, label, and shake. *Keep out of reach of children.*

For a strain or sprain—on the first day do a 15-minute ice pack— then massage the area. Thereafter massage the area three times a day.

basic bath salts

Epsom salt is a good soaking aid for muscle fatigue and drawing out toxins. Milk powder makes the skin soft and silky; but it isn't absolutely necessary. Baking soda softens the water, which in turn softens the skin.

Once prepared, when you smell these, they will seem strong, but remember you will be using a small amount in a tubful of hot water, so they will dissipate. Put about 1/4 cup into the tub as you draw the bath. Relax and indulge yourself. We make this in large quantities to give as gifts. The following recipe makes one 8-ounce jar each and can easily be multiplied for larger quantities.

7/8 cup Epsom salt
About 10 to 12 drops essential oil
2 tablespoons milk powder
2 tablespoons baking soda
Put the salt in a non-reactive container and sprinkle the essential oil over it. Use a spoon to stir it around. Add the milk powder and baking soda and blend well. Pour the salt into a clean jar, cover with a lid and label; *keep out of reach of children*.

Note: An 8-ounce jar is enough for about 3 or 4 baths; when giving this as a gift include these instructions on the label.

Here are two of Susan's most used blends for bath salts, follow the recipe above and use the following essential oil blends:

well body bath salts (cooling, head-clearing, invigorating)

She uses this in the bath for muscle fatigue and tension, after a long hard day, if she has cold or flu symptoms, or needs a boost.

essential oil blend for 1 cup bath salts:
4 to 5 drops eucalyptus
4 to 5 drops rosemary
2 to 3 drops peppermint

bliss blend bath salts (calming, soothing, warming, sensual)

Susan calls this bliss bath because it makes her feel relaxed and blissed out when she gets in the tub. It's calming after a long day and uplifting to the spirit, not to mention sensual.

essential oil blend for 1 cup bath salts:
4 drops lavender
3 drops cedarwood
3 drops clary sage
2 drops chamomile

*Caution: It is not safe to use many essential oils if you are pregnant or nursing, so contact your health care provider if you have any concerns or questions. Keep out of reach of children. Since each individual may react differently, if you have allergies or have not used these particular essential oils before, you should do a **patch test**, which is described in the **definition of terms**.*

bath bags

We use dried herbs, flowers, seeds and peel to make bath bags and tie them up in pieces of muslin or cheesecloth. The small *bouquet garni* bags are ideal for this; they can be emptied, dried and used again. Some favorite combos are lavender leaves and flowers with maybe a few rose petals, lemon herbs with fennel seeds, rose geranium with orange or grapefruit peel, and chamomile and/or calendula petals with lemon peel or lemon herbs. Be creative.

Place the bag in the tub as you draw your bath. We usually add a few drops of almond or sesame oil, not more than a teaspoon, to the water. It softens and lubricates the skin and we find it captures the scent of the bath herbs so that it lingers on your skin.

Use your own home-dried herbs to create unique and fragrant bath blends of your own. For gift giving, pack the herbal bath blends in to a pretty jar, label, and include a little scoop or seashell for measuring the herbs along with a muslin bag to hold the herbs. Include instructions for filling and using the bags and how to prepare the bath.

sugar scrubs

This is not edible—it is for your skin. Sugar cane produces glycolic acid, which is a natural alpha hydroxy acid that exfoliates the skin. This doesn't dry your skin out like a salt scrub does and will leave your skin feeling really soft and well lubricated. Use whatever combination of dried herbs you like—a combination of 2 or 3 is good—remove the leaves or flowers from stems. Essential oils may also be used, just be sure that they are pure oils and not chemically made. This basic recipe fits into an 8-ounce jar.

Vegetable glycerin has anti-fermentative qualities and is mildly antiseptic. It helps, though not indefinitely, to keep ingredients moist, retard oxidation, and preserve volatile oils. The scrub can be made without it; we add it to scrubs when giving them as gifts, although we don't add it to our home scrubs since we use them up so quickly.

In the shower, scoop some scrub into your hand and gently massage it into your skin. Leave for a minute or two and rinse with warm water. Sometimes after using—the sugar gets a bit hard from water getting mixed with it—just rub between your hands to crumble it and use as directed. When the scrub is just about gone, if liquid and herbs remain in the bottom of the jar, add another scoop of sugar & shake the jar.

Caution: Please be careful in shower when using oil, since it may be slippery. Gently pat dry. It is best not to use this for the first time before a special event in case the cleansing causes blotchy skin. Keep out of reach of children.

herb potpourri sugar scrub

This is one of Susan's favorite spa herb treatments. Besides being good for the skin, these herbs are soothing, anti-stressful and uplifting.

Lavender is a cell regenerator and has the reputation for slowing wrinkles. It is used on scarring, burns, sun-damaged skin, stretch marks, rashes and skin infections.
Chamomile is good for all skin types and can be used to treat sensitive or puffy skin as well as rashes and enlarged capillaries.
Calendula heals skin wounds, rashes, inflammations and bites.
Basil is good for oily skin and sore muscles.

1 cup less 2 tablespoons white or brown sugar
2 ounces (about 6 tablespoons) almond, olive, grape seed or jojoba oil or a combination thereof
About 2 tablespoons total: equal parts organic dried lavender blooms, chamomile flowers, calendula petals and basil leaves
a few drops of essential oils of lavender and/or chamomile
1 teaspoon vegetable glycerin, optional

Put the sugar in a non-reactive bowl. If using dried herbs, crush them with a mortar and pestle, or chop them fine and add them to the sugar. If using essential oils for fragrance drop them into the carrier oil to disperse them. Add the glycerin to the oil if using it. Blend well, transfer into clean jars, use plastic lids and label. Keep in a cool place and use within 1 month. *Keep out of reach of children.*

In the shower, scoop some scrub into your hand and gently massage it into your skin. Leave for a minute or two and rinse with warm water.

bliss blend sugar scrub
(calming, soothing, warming, sensual)

1 cup less 2 tablespoons white or brown sugar
2 ounces (about 6 tablespoons) almond, olive, grape seed or jojoba
oil or a combination thereof
bliss blend of essential oils:
4 drops lavender
3 drops each cedarwood and clary sage
2 drops chamomile
1 teaspoon vegetable glycerin, optional

Put the sugar in a non-reactive bowl. Drop the essential oils into
the oil to disperse. Add the oil and glycerin to the sugar. Blend
well, transfer into clean jars, use plastic lids and label. Keep out of
reach of children. Keep in a cool place and use within 1 month.

In the shower, scoop some scrub into your hand and gently
massage it into your skin. Leave for a minute or two and rinse with
warm water.

*Caution: Since each individual may react differently, if you have
allergies or have not used these particular essential oils before, you
should do a skin test by rubbing the scrub on the inner part of your
elbow and waiting a few hours, before using all over your body or
face. It is not safe to use many essential oils if you are pregnant
or nursing, so contact your health care provider if you have any
concerns or questions.*

foot soaks

The simple pleasure of sitting in a comfortable chair with your feet immersed in warm water is a great way to get therapeutic benefit from herbs and essential oils. The body relaxes, skin and toe nail tissues soften and the steam opens the sinuses. This therapy does not require high dollar equipment, though there are all sorts of fun foot-soaking units available on the market. All that is needed is a heat source, a non-reactive pot and a basin large enough to completely submerge the feet in water.

Tina's Granddad Bristow came in from his cotton fields everyday for dinner. That is the country name for the noon day meal. Her grandma, "Two-Mommy" would serve biscuits and sausage left over from breakfast, and cooked vegetables like squash and black-eyed peas and a big glass of buttermilk. For dessert, Granddad would sprinkle salt on the top of his buttermilk and dip soda crackers or cornbread in the glass. Then, he would rise up from the kitchen table and make his way to his rocking chair, take off his boots and open his newspaper.

Two-Mommy would pour some of the water she was heating for washing dishes in a big basin, sprinkle in some Epsom salts, and set the basin down at Granddad's feet. He would read his paper and soak his feet while the radio played old-time Gospel music. After a while, he would stretch out on the bed for a nap. Around mid-afternoon he would walk back out to the fields and labor until dark. Soaking his feet helped Granddad get his work done.

ozark foot soak

Tina uses the herbs in this recipe because they are found around her home. White oak is harvested for weaving baskets and chair bottoms by craftspeople in the Ozark region. It is also cut for firewood. It is easy to find a downed oak branch to whittle for its bark. This harvest method is called "barking." It is not necessary to separate the outer bark from the inner bark when preparing a foot soak. The inner bark contains tannic acid, a substance used to harden leather and makes skin feel soft. Horsemint (Monarda punctata) is native to the Ozarks and is rich in thymol, a very strong antiseptic and anti-fungal essential oil. Mint and jewelweed grow abundantly near springs and are prolific if planted in the garden. Mint cools and stimulates the feet. The juice of fresh jewelweed helps stop itching and speeds the healing of rashes and bites. Comfrey is easy to grow in the garden. It contains allantoin that speeds the healing of sprains and bruises. This preparation is both a decoction and an infusion.

2 gallons water
1 small handful white oak bark strips
1 bunch horsemint
1 bunch dried mint (spearmint or peppermint varieties)
4 to 7 dried comfrey leaves
1 cup jewelweed vinegar

Place the water and bark into a large non-reactive pan. Cover and bring to a boil; simmer 20 minutes. Meanwhile, crush the herbs with a mortar and pestle or chop them coarsely. Turn off the heat and add the herbs. Cover and steep for 10 minutes or so.

Pour the mixture into a wide and shallow foot soak pan. Add enough cool water to bring the water to a comfortable temperature. Soak the feet for as long as it feels nice. You can add a little more hot water if it starts to cool down and you aren't ready to get up. Massaging the feet enhances this pleasurable experience. When ready, pat the feet dry with a soft towel.

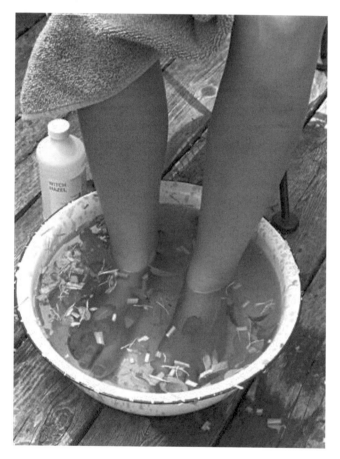

an herbal foot soak is one of the most relaxing things you can do for yourself or someone you love

city folk foot soak

This is an alternative to the Ozark version because the ingredients are available in stores. Lemongrass is fragrant, calming and most importantly, an anti-fungal for athlete's foot and ringworm. Green tea contains tannic acid in place of the white oak bark. Witch hazel is available in the pharmacy to treat minor skin irritation. In place of comfrey, arnica ointment may be kept on hand to treat bruises and/or achy joints. Sometimes, we let the "soakee" choose a fragrant essential oil from our collection and drop in a few drops just before soaking. Susan likes to add petals from a few fresh or dried calendula flowers.

2 gallons water
1 cup dried or 2 cups fresh lemongrass leaves
3 green tea bags or about 1 generous tablespoon green tea leaves
3 mint tea bags (spearmint or peppermint) or about 1 generous tablespoon mint leaves
1/2 cup witch hazel astringent

Bring the water to a boil in a large, non-reactive pan. Turn off the heat. Add the tea bags or loose tea, cover, and steep for 10 minutes. Pour the infusion into a wide shallow foot-soak pan. Soak the feet for as long as it feels nice. When ready, pat the feet dry with a soft towel

Eating homemade chocolate pudding or drinking an herbal libation even further enhances the foot-soak experience.

beauty toe

For years, Susan and her daughters, Lucie and Cady, and the women in her family have practiced a female ritual called "beauty toe". Like many women and girls throughout the ages, this is time set aside to pamper physical and emotional bodies. The preparation is part of the fun of the whole experience. Tasty snacks and beverages are prepared. A big pot of water is brought to a simmer and the herbs and essential oils are chosen. Toenail clippers, files, nail buffers, almond oil and soft towels are assembled. Favorite music is played. Amidst giggles and serious conversation, each person has their turn at beauty toe.

First, the feet are soaked with an essential oil fragrance of choice, then the toenails are trimmed and manicured. Next the fortunate one reclines on plumped pillows with an eye mask, if desired. While massaging oil into one another's feet—tenderness soothes the spirit and the whole experience is nurturing—a balm that heals the soul and soles. Of course if you are up for it, you can choose your favorite color of nail polish, which completes the beauty-toe treatment.

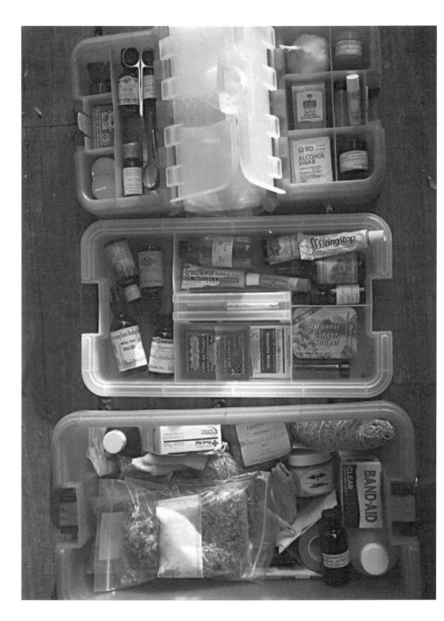

herbal home remedy kit: three-tiered toolbox

herbal kits

In the seventh grade, Susan had to make a first-aid kit for her science class project. It was not very big and was rather basic: band-aids, first aid cream, gauze, sticky white tape, scissors, iodine, and a few other items. Having been a Girl Scout, she had to earn a first-aid badge and had to learn about first aid, as well as making a splint and tying a *tourniquet*. Growing up, she didn't have a so-called first-aid kit in her home, because everything was in the medicine cabinet, but there was one at her grandparents' shore house and onboard the boat, along with a fire extinguisher. As a young adult, headed across country, she had a store-bought Johnson & Johnson® plastic-boxed kit under the front seat of the car.

Over the years, both Susan and Tina Marie's ideas of first aid have changed quite a bit. Being a parent, Susan did have a bottle of syrup of Ipecac on hand (to induce vomiting in case of poisoning). There are basic standard ingredients in our kits today as there were back when we were young, but many of our remedies have changed with the times and our continuing herbal education. Over the years, we have learned to make poultices, salves, tinctures, teas and synergistic blends of herbs and essential oils. Susan's herbal apprenticeship with Rosemary Gladstar, the Science and Art of Herbalism, was an amazing learning experience with medicinal herbs and prompted her to make an herbal home remedy kit.

Susan had herbal products that she had been making in all parts of the house from the pantry, cold room, office and bedroom, to the bathroom and the kids' bathroom. So she decided to put it together and contain it all in one place. Once, she began gathering the ingredients and supplies, she realized that she needed a container to store it all in and that sent her on a search for the perfect box. She looked at art boxes, fishing tackle boxes, cosmetic boxes, sewing boxes, and finally settled on a heavy-duty plastic toolbox with three tiers. Things get taken out of it and eventually find their way back. Items are still sort of all over the place—since she has some around the house, in the car and her travel kit—however, she keeps most of the remedy kit together in one place. It is important that everything in your remedy kit be labeled, and even better if you have an instruction sheet as to what each item is used for.

The Girl Scouts' motto is "Be prepared"—and we are with our very own herbal home remedy kits. Below is a list of what is in Susan's kit; it is what she uses and what works best for her family. Tina Marie's kit is different from Susan's, yet has many of the same ingredients. What works for us, may not work for you; we hope this will inspire you to create your own **herbal remedy kit**.

The information here does not intend to treat, diagnose or prescribe and therefore does not take responsibility for your experience in using these remedies. Contact your health care practitioner if you have questions, if you are on prescription drugs, or if you are pregnant or nursing.

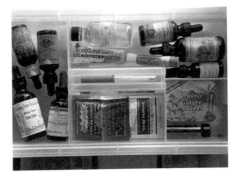

close-up of ingredients in herbal remedy kit

herbal home remedy kit

assorted standard ingredients
These items are fairly standard items to have on hand in any first-aid kit.

bandages—assorted sizes
band-aids®—variety of sizes; decorative ones are especially good for small children
scissors
thermometer
tweezers
magnifying glass
needles/safety pins—all sizes
matches
candles
hot water bottle
ice bag
alcohol swabs
toothpicks/natural floss

supplies and ingredients
The following are items in Susan's herbal home remedy kit.

clean, washed muslin or cotton cheesecloth (if you don't wash it first the sizing of the fabric makes it difficult for absorption; also it makes it softer and less stiff)—to use as a compress or for wrapping wounds and poultices.

wool socks or sweater sleeves—these are perfect for holding poultices or bandages in place without using tape and they hold fast; just slide them over the arm, elbow, ankle or leg. They also tend to hold heat.

vetwrap—this stretchy and flexible wrap sticks to itself, so it is perfect for wrapping wounds or holding poultices. It comes in a roll and can be purchased at pet stores and feed stores that deal in animal products. We've recently found similar products at the drugstore sold as sports wrap.

moleskin—there is nothing like soft and flexible moleskin made from cotton flannel for wrapping any tender spot—a toe or parts of the foot (ballerinas can't live without it—they stuff their toe shoes—neither can teenage girls with new shoes)—for protection from shoes or boots that have rubbed a blister. You can wrap the sore area entirely, or you can cut the moleskin and make a circle surrounding the blister, which is elevated and holds anything from touching the blister.

eyecup—an indispensable tool for washing or rinsing the eye; when Susan was a kid her family had a cobalt blue glass eyecup on a little pedestal like a wineglass, however nowadays the glass ones are hard to find; we have seen them occasionally in antique stores in pale pink, pale green, or clear glass. They can be found at the local pharmacy but they are made of plastic.

tea strainer or tea ball—these are handy for making tea, an infusion or decoction, especially if you don't have a strainer and you need a clear liquid. They are also handy to have to heat herbs or bark for a poultice.

Rescue Remedy ®—this product is a Bach flower remedy—and is described as one of the world's best known natural stress relief remedies. It is made from a combination of five flower essences: cherry plum, clematis, impatiens, rock rose, and Star of Bethlehem and 27% alcohol. We use this whenever we hurt ourselves, or feel very emotional due to a lot of stress, bad news, are in shock or am feeling panic. We have used Rescue Remedy on ourselves for more than 20 years. We keep it in the house, in the car, and take it when we travel.

spritzers—We make spritzers from distilled water and essential oils and put them in cobalt blue bottles with mist sprayers. We have different blends that we use for their aromatherapeutic properties, as well as their anti-bacterial qualities. We keep them all over the house, in the car, and our travel bags.

aloe vera gel—is the most soothing of remedies for sunburn, and we also use it for minor kitchen burns and to soothe rashes. We break off or cut a piece of our plants and rub the clear, gel-like sap right onto the skin. We also keep a bottle of aloe vera gel in the refrigerator to have on hand for making herbal products. Caution: Aloe should never be used on a staph infection as it will seal in the bacteria, allowing it to multiply.

powdered clay—We keep green powdered clay on hand to use for cleansing facials every now and then, but mostly we keep it in powdered form in little jars—one in our home remedy kit and one in our travel kit—because of its drawing ability. Whenever we have a splinter or a thorn that is hard to get, we mix a little clay with water and put it on the area; as the clay dries it draws out the culprit. It is drawing and drying when used as a poultice.

witch hazel—this astringent can be used as a disinfectant to clean skin, used on minor irritations, relieves itching, and as a liniment for sore muscles.

lip balm—for chapped lips

green salve—there are many variations of green salves—you can buy all-purpose ones from the health food store—they are used for insect bites, skin irritations, minor scrapes and cuts, and chafing.

We make our own using different herbs for specific conditions.

external liniment—We use Jethro Kloss' recipe made from alcohol, myrrh, golden seal, and cayenne; see Back to Eden, Benedict Lust Publications, 1971 for the exact recipe. It can be used as a sore muscle rub and to dry poison ivy. Caution: His recipe is very potent, so we tend to dilute it; try a little skin test on the inside of you elbow to see how it feels on your skin—definitely dilute it if using it on a child, elder, or someone with sensitive skin.

slippery elm lozenges—slippery elm's demulcent properties coat the throat, so these lozenges are soothing for a sore mouth or throat; they come in a number of flavors and taste pleasant. If you take too many of them they will loosen you up on the other end, so don't overdo.

wild cherry syrup—for coughs and sore throat—Susan keeps this on hand for her kids when they can't sleep at night due to coughing, the bark of the wild cherry is an expectorant.

candied ginger—We like candied ginger for an upset tummy or if we overeat; it works good for motion sickness from car, plane or boat, (so Susan keeps it in the car and uses it on airplanes.)

Emer'gen-C®—these little packets are in my pantry, remedy kit, glove compartment, and my carry-on since they are a "super energy booster" and a quick source of vitamin C with 32 mineral complexes when mixed with water—we use them especially in the summer when sweating a lot and when we feel shaky from not eating and need something quick.

arnica gel—even though we make our own arnica oil, we keep a tube of this on hand. It really works when applied to bruises, muscle aches and pains. Applied to a bump immediately, it will often stop bruising; do not use arnica on an open cut, wound or scrape—only on the skin around it.

jewelweed vinegar—Susan learned this recipe from Tina Marie, who uses it to fend off all sorts of biting insects in the Ozarks, and she is now a believer. To make this, infuse jewelweed (Impatiens capensis) in organic apple cider vinegar, add some insect-repellent essential oils if desired—we keep a spray bottle of it by the backdoor all summer—we spray it on poison ivy (helps to dry it up) and bug bites and apply it before going into the woods. See gardening comforts chapter for the recipe.)

garlic—We eat garlic everyday for its many medicinal properties. It will sting when you rub a raw clove of cut garlic on a small boo-boo, but its antiseptic qualities work wonders.

chocolate—whether your injury or hurt is physical or emotional, the natural serotonin in dark chocolate will help make you feel better, and take your mind off of your boo-boo, at least for a brief moment.

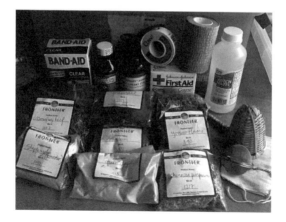

dried herbs are ingredients in our herbal remedy kit

dried herbs

We keep these handy for making herbal infusions. Replace dried herbs with fresh dried herbs annually.

chamomile—used for soothing, calms stress; aids digestion.
comfrey—use ground root and/or leaves externally for poultices for bruises, sprains or strains, and bone injuries.
lemon balm—soothes digestive tract; helps to relax and sleep.
milky oats—the seeds of this plant increase vitality and are a good-tasting tea for relief of stress and anxiety.
peppermint or spearmint—for soothing stomach and to freshen breath.
sage—good for mouth and throat gargle.

tea blends

You can purchase prepared blends manufactured by Traditional Medicinals ® under the names in italics, or something similar from other herbal tea companies, or you can mix up your own blends for specific complaints. Replace dried herbs with fresh dried herbs annually.

colds and lungs—'*Gypsy Cold Care ®*', elder, mullein, yarrow
digestion—mint, fennel
nerve sedatives—chamomile, hops, lemon balm, passionflower, valerian
sore throats—'*Throat Coat ®*', slippery elm, ginger, cherry bark, licorice
traveler's aid—'*Smooth Move ®*', slippery elm, senna, ground flax seed or flax seed oil capsules

powdered herbs

Powdered herbs can be packed in caps, used in poultices or dissolved in tea.

echinacea—boosts the immune system, good for colds and flu, use capsules if you don't prefer the tincture.
slippery elm—for sore throats, scalded tongues or mouth, digestive complaints, constipation.
goldenseal—powdered root is prepared in poultices for infections and abscesses; do not use for more than 2 to 3 weeks at a time since goldenseal irritates mucous membranes.
cayenne—use sparingly since it is very hot; it is a warming stimulating powder, good for the circulation and the heart, as well as digestion and congestion.
yarrow—dried leaves should be powdered to be used on cuts to stop bleeding and disinfect wounds. Rosemary Gladstar recommends placing a pinch in the nose to stop a nosebleed.

tinctures

Tinctures act much more quickly for me than powdered capsules. Since most are made with alcohol, they should not be given to children. Alcohol-free tinctures made with glycerin can be prepared at home or purchased.

echinacea *(Echinacea purpurea)*—for the immune system, colds and flu, infections.
echinacea and goldenseal *(Hydrastis canadensis)*—used for the immune system and to fight infection.
ashwaganda *(Withania somnifera)*—promotes well being; good for low energy.

kava-kava coconut *(Piper methysticum)*—kava is good for calming stress and anxiety; allows the body to relax while the mind stays alert; the coconut milk makes it taste delicious and the fat in the coconut milk helps the kava to be more readily absorbed. *Caution: Kava is a controversial substance, since it can alter one's state of mind; we personally use it carefully since there are warnings about possible liver toxicity.*
crampbark *(Viburnum opulus)*—very good for menstrual cramps.
valerian *(Valeriana officinalis)*—for relaxing, insomnia, stress and tension, relieves aches and pain. *Caution: Some particularly sensitive individuals may have the opposite reaction to valerian— do not use if you feel agitated or uneasy after trying it.*

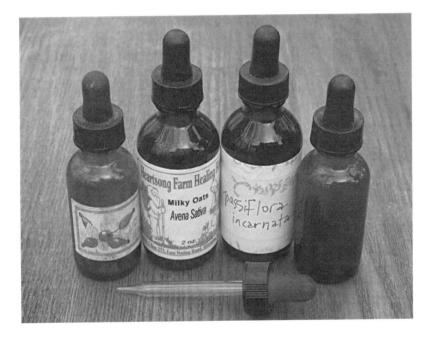

hand-crafted tinctures

essential oils

Most essential oils should not be used 'neat'—they should be diluted. Be sure your oils are pure oils and not synthetically made.

lavender—if we could have only one essential oil it would be lavender. It relieves pain, burns and bee stings, and is superb used in the bath and aromatherapy for relaxation. Inhalation of the steam helps with headaches.

tea tree—has antiseptic, antibiotic, and anti-fungal properties, we use it on cuts and wounds, insect bites, rashes, and for cleansing purposes. A skin test is recommended before using it neat.

eucalyptus—we keep this on hand for baths for achy muscles or cold and flu-like symptoms, use it for a steam inhalation for coughs and congestion, and mixed into our insect repellents.

thyme—another anti-microbial and antiseptic oil, we use it diluted for cleansing purposes, on bites and stings, in the bath for muscle aches, colds and flu; it is also good for bad breath and infections in the mouth.

oils

The following are carrier oils, or oils blended with herbs or essential oils that are used for specific ailments.

arnica oil—for bruises and muscle aches.

calendula oil—soothing to the skin for most minor irritations, bruises, good for dry skin, regenerates cell growth.

castor oil—for swelling and contusions; very drawing as it pulls out toxins (will stain clothing and skin).

mullein flower oil—for earaches.

herbal salve

Basic salve recipes use about 1 cup oil to 1/4 cup beeswax; this gives you a soft salve. To test the consistency, dip a metal spoon into the heated salve, place the spoon in the fridge and check it after a few minutes to see if it is firm and about the right consistency. If you want it a little firmer—add a little more beeswax—to make it softer increase the oil slightly.

We use the following salve for dry rough skin and skin conditions that plague the gardener. We use calendula oil (page 121) since we have had successful results using it on chapped lips, hands and heels, and in massage oils. We also prepare chickweed oil (use the same method as for calendula oil using dried chickweed instead) since it soothes skin discomforts and is abundant in our gardens and yard. This salve can be prepared with just almond or olive oil and calendula oil. The vitamin E oil is optional; it helps prevent oils from becoming rancid so it prolongs the shelf life. EOs are optional—lavender and chamomile are nice in this salve.

Makes about 6 liquid ounces; fills four 1 1/2-ounce containers

1/4 cup calendula oil
1/4 cup chickweed oil
3 packed tablespoons grated natural beeswax
2 teaspoons vitamin E oil, optional
5 to 6 drops essential oil, optional

Heat the combined oils in a saucepan over the lowest heat possible. Add beeswax to the warm oil and stir until melted. Test for consistency. Remove from heat and stir in the EOs and/or vitamin E oil, if desired. Immediately pour the salve into clean containers, let cool without lids; put lids on once completely cool and label.

susan's essential travel kit

The following items are in Susan's travel bag, which accompanies her on every trip that she takes. She has found that by using these essentials, she is more comfortable and stays much healthier.

1. **water**—must have for hydrating when traveling.
2. **spritzers**—to help kill germs in public places; uplift, relax, or stimulate; to refresh stale air in hotel rooms or meeting places.
3. **essential oils**—lavender, tea tree and eucalyptus.
4. **tinctures**—echinacea and valerian.
5. **candles**—soothing and well-being.
6. **natural incense and matches**—for changing the atmosphere and air-quality of a hotel room.
7. **Basic H ™ or Dr. Bronner's Castile Soap**—surfactant cleaners.
8. **apple cider vinegar with tea tree oil**—keep this in a spritzer-type bottle and use for spritzing the shower/bathtub of a public place or hotel room to kill germs and make it possible to take a bath without the fear of getting cooties.
9. **bath oil or bubble bath**—for relaxing and de-stressing while traveling.
10. **lotion**—for moisturizing dry skin.
11. **herbal salve**—for itches or scrapes.
12. **lip balm**—for moisturizing lips.
13. **Tiger Balm®**—for headaches or stuffy heads and chest.
14. **Rescue Remedy®**—natural stress relief.
15. **herb tea bags, Emer'gen-C®**--restoratives, digestives, etc.
16. **candied ginger**—for motion sickness and indigestion.
17. **arnica gel or oil**—for bruises, swelling and joint stiffness.
18. **three essential foods** for everyday and emergencies:
    chocolate
    garlic
    chile peppers

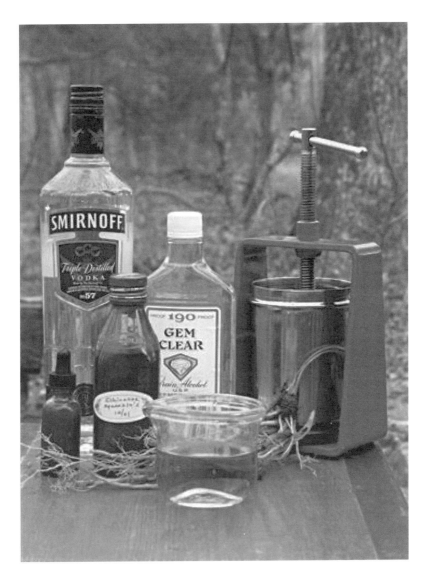

tincture-making supplies: alcohol for the menstruum, echinacea root, tincture press, mortar and pestle, dark glass tincture bottles

tinctures

We have been making tinctures for home use for many years.
The first one Tina ever made was with Steven Foster during her
herbal apprenticeship for the Ozark Folk Center's Heritage Herb
Garden. The botanical was passionflower (*Passiflora incarnata*),
harvested during one of many herbal odysseys of that propitious
year. The entire vine, including the stems, leaves and unripe fruit
was chopped, placed in a mason jar and covered with vodka. It was
left to macerate for one month. It was then filtered and poured into
a labeled, brown glass bottle. Steven required Tina to research the
uses for herb. She learned that it has historical uses with modern
day credibility. Extracts of *Passiflora* are taken as a nervine to
reduce anxiety in Europe. Passionflower tincture, added to hot
milk, has helped Tina get to sleep on more than one restless night.
It was empowering to learn how easy it is to tincture plants so that
they are handy when needed.

Chaste tree (*Vitex agnus-castus*) seed tincture came was helpful
for both of us as we transitioned through the hot flashes and other
special effects of menopause. We stripped the seed from our
respective shrubs during the fall, crushed them with a mortar and
pestle and macerated them in a menstruum of silver label vodka.
The knowledge of that herb and a host of other green allies serve
us well. The process filled a need to take positive, self-sufficient
action while our bodies, emotions and spirits went through natural
changes. Susan also tinctured black cohosh (*Cimicifuga racemosa)*
to great benefit during those years.

We each make a supply of echinacea tincture every year and a
quart of passionflower is put away nearly every season. New
tinctures are dreamed up according to what herbs we are studying

as time goes by. The International Herb Association's Herb of the Year program has inspired lemon balm, oregano, rosemary and thyme tinctures. Garlic tincture wasn't as pleasant as some made with other Herbs of the Year. We have also tinctured calendula flowers, valerian, kava, hawthorn berries, and made a rose glycerite. Sometimes tincturing is a way to use an herb that needs pruning on a particular day. Our apothecaries grow right along with our knowledge of plants.

Although we often use herbs synergistically, we tincture them separately and then blend them as needed. We probably use silver label vodka and Everclear most often; however, Susan likes the flavor of rum and brandy. Tina tested moonshine as a menstruum and it was pretty smooth.

growing our own medicinal coneflowers

We cultivate all the species of echinacea because they are handsome perennial flowering plants that add height and color to our gardens, and show off their splendid cone heads throughout the summer and into the fall. Butterflies and birds are attracted to these bright purple-pink, pale lavender, white, and yellow coneflowers.

During the flowering season and again, after the plants go dormant in the colder weather, we reap the health benefits by harvesting the plants and making our own tinctures. When we prepare them with our own organically grown plants, they are truly the best.

conservation

Most commercial *E. pallida* and *E. angustifolia* tinctures are made with wild-crafted plants. There are some promising developments in the field cultivation of these two echinacea species. We are concerned for the declining wild populations of these species because of the global demand for echinacea products and human pressures on their natural habitats. On the bright side, most of the plants used to make *E. purpurea* tincture are cultivated. When we have to purchase echinacea tincture we look for the words "organically grown *Echinacea purpurea*" on the label. The herbalist's vow is to do no harm. This includes protecting the native populations and habitats of our herbs.

Another way herbal consumers can participate in the conservation of native populations of echinacea is by growing our own plants and making our own tinctures. This is as grounding and fulfilling as growing our own food. Our harvesting methods actually enhance the health of our plants.

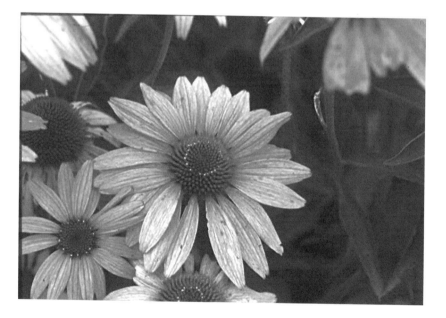

*purple coneflowers are easy to grow and medicine can be
made from the flowers, leaves & root*

harvesting echinacea tops

Leaves and flowers can be selectively pruned and tinctured in the summer. This practice prolongs blooming and increases the air circulation around the plants. The plants selected for tincturing should at least be in their second year of growth. Allow them to establish a good root system with undisturbed leaf growth the first year. With a light hand and the intent to leave the plants in good shape, harvest flowering stems as if you were making a bouquet. Cut the stems above a node or at the crown. See the instructions for preparing the herbs and making the tincture below. Echinacea tops are macerated for only 48 hours.

harvesting echinacea roots

In this section, we begin by harvesting the echinacea root to take you through the tincture-making process from start to finish.

As echinacea ages, clumps are formed with new plants sprouting around the original plant. The oldest plants in the clump may decline as the younger vigorous plants compete for nutritional resources. Dividing the clumps regenerates the plants and gives a perfect opportunity to harvest roots for tincture. For root tincturing, we choose plants that are at least three years old.

We harvest echinacea roots by digging a circle one and one-half to two feet out from the drip line of the plant. Sink the tool deeply; we use a fork, but a shovel works. The idea is to harvest as much root as possible. The roots grow deep and extend out in a wide perimeter around the crown.

Keep the crowns of the plants intact with the roots so that it will be easy to identify the echinacea from the roots of neighboring plants. Tracing the roots from the crown is a sure way to learn the differences in underground parts.

Shake and massage the soil and unwanted plant roots from the clump. This is a good time to kill a few weeds. Leave as much soil as possible in the garden.

It is best to harvest and tincture on the same day.

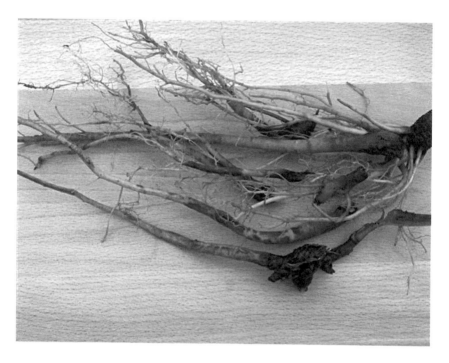

just-harvested echinacea root

preparing the echinacea roots

Once harvested, we carefully separate the plants from the clump. The first thing we do is decide which new shoots to put aside for replanting and carefully trim the roots for tincture, leaving enough intact for the plant to survive. Then we trim roots from the crowns that we will replant. Once this is done it is important to loosely wrap the plants and crowns in damp paper towels and put them into plastic bags so that they don't dry out. They will keep this way, for a few days if necessary, until we can replant them. However, we like to get them back into the earth as soon as possible.

Next comes the washing process. Scrub larger roots with a brush and rinse and rub the thinner, fibrous roots to be sure to remove any grit. Place all of the washed roots in a colander to drain.

Separate the larger roots from the finer ones. A heavy-duty sharp knife and wooden cutting board are essential for chopping the large, thick, hard stems. Slice big roots crosswise into rounds (as if cutting carrots) and then chop them into smaller pieces. Once chopped, put them aside and chop the finer roots coarsely.

details on making the tincture

We use a large pharmaceutical porcelain mortar and pestle to pound the echinacea root. Begin with the larger root pieces, using the pestle to crush them. This takes a little bit of time, but it is pleasant work. Add a little of the menstruum to the roots, to help with the pounding if necessary. Once the hard woody pieces are pretty well mashed, remove them and add the smaller roots. Make a mash out of these and then combine all of the roots.

A menstruum is the liquid used to extract the soluble principles from the herbs or roots. It can be alcohol, vinegar or vegetable glycerin for a non-alcoholic tincture. We use 90- or 100-proof vodka, which provides the proper ratio of water to alcohol. A combination of both alcohol (at least 25 %) and water is needed to extract all of the constituents from the herbs. If we use Everclear which is a pure grain alcohol at 190 proof, we dilute it with half distilled water. You can use another alcohol like rum, brandy or gin, if you prefer.

Measure and transfer the pounded root into a clean glass jar with a plastic lid. The ratio of echinacea root to menstruum is 1 to 2. If there is 1 cup of root, add 2 cups of menstruum. Put the lid on the jar and label it with the date. We shake our tincture twice daily—in the morning—and the evening. Leave the tincture for 2 to 6 weeks. We prefer to leave our tinctures for the longer amount of time.

Above-ground plant parts (leaves, flowers and/or stems) should be washed and pounded, just like the roots. They are infused for only 48 hours, because, after that time, the beneficial compounds begin to decompose.

When the tincture is ready, strain it through a strainer lined with fine cheesecloth, or we find that a yogurt cheese maker is ideal for this. Mash down on the roots to extract every last bit of tincture from them. Alternatively, a tincture press this job is made easy.

Tinctures should be stored in dark glass bottles in a cool place, away from light. We save bottles for this purpose and we pick up new rubber droppers at the health food store for our tincture bottles, since the rubber tends to disintegrate with age. Be sure to label your tinctures and date them.

echinacea root tincture

Please read tincture-making details above before you start.
Echinacea has been used medicinally for centuries by Native
Americans to combat many ailments. It is believed that echinacea
stimulates the immune system and its anti-viral activities help fight
colds and flu, as well as promote healing of infections.

Our years of personal experience of using the tincture is that it
keeps us healthier by helping us to avoid colds and flu, decreases
the duration and severity of these symptoms, and helps our
bodies fight infections. We take echinacea tincture during the
cold and flu season, at the first signs of a cold or when we are
fighting an infection, and especially when we travel and are
around large groups of people. The tincture can be taken straight
by the dropperful or diluted in water. Or, its earthy, rather
medicinal taste can be disguised in fruit juice. We also apply the
tincture topically to inflammations such as hangnails, bug bites
and toothaches.

Caution: Those with impaired immune systems should consult with
their health care practitioner before using immuno-stimulants.
Since echinacea is a member of the aster/daisy family, which
ragweed is a relative; some individuals may be allergic to it.

1 cup fresh echinacea roots, scrubbed, chopped and ground
1 cup 190 proof ethanol alcohol (Everclear) and 1 cup distilled
water OR 2 cups vodka (90 to 100 proof)

Place prepared roots in a clean jar. Cover with the menstruum of
alcohol and water. Keep in a cool dark place. Shake twice daily.
Macerate for 2 to 6 weeks. Filter the tincture through unbleached
paper coffee filter. Pour the finished tincture into a brown glass
bottle and label.

tincturing by percolation

The evolution of herbal studies has led us to tincturing by percolation. James Green, in *The Herbal Medicine Maker's Handbook: A Home Manual*, devotes an entire chapter to the subject. A simplified explanation of this fascinating method of tincturing may be enough to whet the curiosity of folks interested in making very high-quality tinctures. There is a bit more calculation, measuring and attention to detail to get successful results with the "perc cone"; however, it is a very exciting process with a great end result.

In essence, the percolation method extracts the soluble properties of the herb by slowly passing the chosen menstruum through a column of freshly dried, powdered herb. The process works by means of gravity and the movement of displaced, charged molecules of solvent from the herb. As molecules of the solvent are charged with the plant chemicals, they move downward and out of the way and are replaced by new, uncharged solvent molecules from above.

The process requires a special glass percolation cone, a stand, tubing and a clamp to fit the tubing. The desired dried herb is weighed, pre-moistened and methodically packed into the cone. The menstruum is carefully poured over the herb and the complete extraction of the herb's properties is accomplished in about 24 hours. When the tincture is drained off, the marc (herb) is nearly colorless and has lost its aroma, smelling only of the menstruum. The resulting solution is quite strong and uniform in color.

When Susan read of this tincturing method she was inspired, and so she went online in search. After a few dead ends, she found Richard McDonald at www.desertbloomherbs.com and learned many details on tincturing by the percolation method from him. This eventually led her to Allen Scientific Glass, Inc. allenglass@cmonline.com where she ordered a handmade glass 2-liter percolation cone. She ended up ordering the hardware apparatus (rod, support stand, ring support, and clamp) from Science Kit & Boreal Laboratories at http://www.sciencekit.com and eventually found the right hose and clamp at a local wine-making shop. We are now able to make large quantities of tincture in about 24 hours.

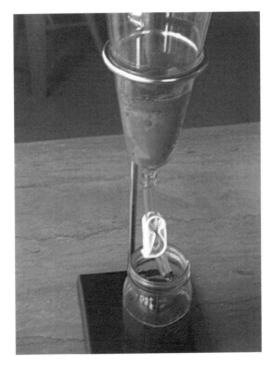

percolation cone with leftover marc and
finished tincture in jar

the science of tincturing

Tinctures are preserved plant extracts made with diluted alcohol or glycerin. Tincturing is accomplished by two methods, percolation and maceration. Percolation requires expensive lab equipment.

Tincture strength is expressed as a weight/volume ratio. Plant material is weighed in grams. Menstruum is measured in liters. The standards for tincture were created in 1902 and called the International Protocol.

A 10% tincture (1:10 w/v) uses dried toxic or intense herb at a rate of 10 grams of herb to 100 cc of menstruum.

A 20% tincture (1:5 w/v) uses dried non-toxic herb at a rate of 20 grams of herb to 100 cc of menstruum.

A 50% tincture (1:2 w/v) uses 50 grams of fresh herb to 100 cc of menstruum. Fresh herb tinctures are often made with 100% grain alcohol.

Maceration is done in a sealed glass vessel. Dried or fresh plant material is triturated (finely crushed or chopped) and covered with the menstruum. The tincture is shaken frequently (twice a day).

Duration of the process varies, depending upon the herbalist. A minimum of 14 days is suggested. To finish, decant and filter the solution. Press the marc. Filter the resulting liquid. Combine the two liquids. Store finished tincture in a tightly sealed glass container away from heat. Shake before taking.

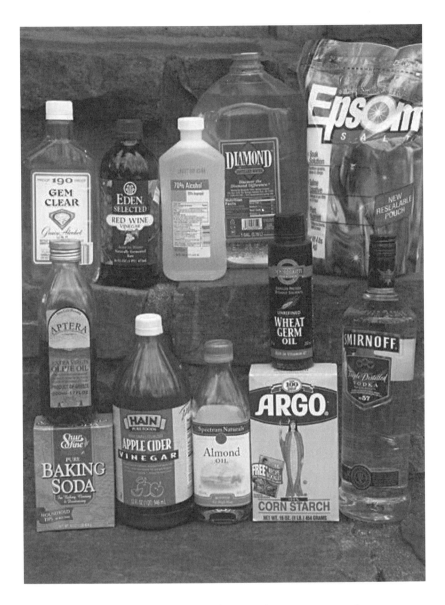

*common household ingredients are used
in the creative herbal home*

ingredients

Alcohol, either rubbing (isopropyl) or grain (ethyl), is an antiseptic solvent that evaporates quickly. *Caution: Rubbing alcohol must never be taken internally.*

Ethyl alcohol, which is also called grain alcohol, is used for making tinctures. Alcohol extracts essential oils, alkaloids, resins and glycosides. Alcohol halts the destruction of alkaloids and glycosides by enzymes. By eliminating microbial activity, alcohol preserves plant material almost indefinitely. Alcohol does not dissolve undesired gums, albumins and starches.

Grain alcohol is 190 proof or 95% alcohol or 151 proof or 75.5% alcohol. Distilled water is added to grain alcohol to dilute it to the desired percentage appropriate to the herb being extracted (see the **science of tincturing**.) Vodka or rum is generally 80 proof or 40% alcohol or 90 proof (look for the silver label) at 45% alcohol. These can usually be used without further dilution. Tinctures are also made with wine and brandy.

We use rubbing (isopropyl) alcohol as a carrier for essential oils to make fast-drying cleaning agents for books, fabrics and glass. Alcohol is a solvent that can dissolve bandage adhesives for painless removal. It will kill mold, mildew, germs and remove vomit stains. It is good for cleaning razor blades, scissors and pruning shears by cutting residue and drying quickly, thereby preventing rust. Alcohol sprayed on wasps with a trigger sprayer will kill them. Make soft, malleable ice packs for bruises and muscle aches by freezing equal parts water and alcohol in a plastic bag. Vodka can be used in place of rubbing alcohol for these purposes.

Baking soda or bicarbonate of soda is a naturally occurring mineral. It is a gentle abrasive for cleaning hard surfaces, is absorbent and neutralizes odors and acids.

Beeswax is heated and combined with fats to make salves and lip balm. The result is a semi-solid substance that melts at body temperature. Beeswax will smell like honey when fresh. The very best source is comes from local hives. Contact your state extension office for beekeepers near your home or shop at the local farmers' market. Local honey may be sold there and farmers, especially fruit growers, will know the beekeepers. Alternatively, purchase honey with the honeycomb in the jar. Pour the contents of the jar through a sieve to catch the wax. Leave until all the honey has dripped out. Then, put the honey back in the jar. Boil the beeswax in water until the wax melts. Remove from heat and allow the water to cool. The wax will rise to the top. Break into pieces, dry it completely and store in a dark glass jar.

Castile soap is a blend of plant-based surfactants for all-purpose cleaning applications. There are many companies making liquid castile soap and castile soap in a bar. One of the oldest manufacturers is Dr. Bronner's; their liquid, Pure-Castile Soap comes unscented or with essential oils already added. It can be used for everything from washing dishes or vegetables to lingerie, your body or teeth. Dr. Bronner's Sal Suds is stronger than castile soap and is used for household cleaner; it contains the essential oils of spruce and fir. See **surfactant** for more info.

Castor oil is expressed from the seed of the castor bean plant (*Ricinus communis*). The oil is used as a laxative and a lubricating agent in soaps and cosmetics. The seed contains the deadly toxins ricinine and ricin. The oil does not contain these toxins but overdose can cause vomiting.

Cocoa butter, chocolate, and **cocoa** come from the fermented, dried and roasted seed of the plant, *Theobroma cacao*. Cocoa butter is solid at normal room temperature and melts at body temperature. This characteristic lends its self well to emollient and delicious lip balm formulations, though the balm will melt if you carry it in your pocket. Cocoa butter is really fatty — it is lubricating, not moisturizing — it is great for dry skin, but not for oily. Store them at room temperature in a cool place, out of direct light

Cornstarch is made by grinding the white hearts of corn kernels to powder. It is absorbent and non-irritating to the skin when used as a powder.

Epsom salts, chemically speaking, is magnesium sulfate. The first Epsom salts were made by boiling down mineral waters from a spring located in Epsom, England. They have been extracted from seawater. Now Epsom salts are mined from limestone cave walls and salt lake deposits.

Essential oils or **EOs** — see chapter on **essential oils**.

Glycerin is a triatomic alcohol and the sweet principle of oils. It is a by-product of soap making. When fixed oils are heated with water and alkalis (lye), the oil forms soap. Synthetic glycerin is made by heating a petroleum product (trichlorpropane) with water. We would rather make tinctures with vegetable glycerin.

Glycerites are extracts (tinctures) made with pure glycerin and fresh plant material, water/glycerin solutions, or alcohol tinctures with glycerin added. Vegetable glycerin has some very good preservative qualities. A properly made glycerite tincture will have a shelf life of up to three years. Glycerin will bind with plant tannins and keep them from precipitating with alkaloids.

Herbs see chapter on **herbs**.

Honey is an ancient remedy for healing infected sores and wounds. Clinical studies suggest that honey is anti-microbial. That action is increased when the honey is diluted with water, which produces hydrogen peroxide. We found this information several places on the Web. The honey Web site, www.hythes.com explained it as follows. An Australian researcher, Shoan Blair, from the University of Sidney found that when raw honey is applied to a wound, the enzyme, glucose oxidase, which is produced by bees, reacts with the water in the wound and the glucose in the honey. Hydrogen peroxide is produced and infections are discouraged because the bacteria cannot grow. Currently, honey is used to treat a wide range of skin infections including staph infections and diabetic sores. Consumption of honey from local hives is thought by some health food advocates to be a way to reduce seasonal allergy symptoms.

Honey contains about 60 percent more sucrose than white sugar. Babies under the age of two should not be given honey in any form because of the risk of death associated with botulism (Clostridium botulinum).

Hydrogen peroxide, chemically expressed as H_2O_2, is anti-microbial and is great for removing bloodstains from fabrics. Hydrogen peroxide, diluted to 3% is readily available at drug and grocery stores (see **washing salads** in **household preparations** for information on hydrogen peroxide and the E. coli bacteria).

Lotion (fragrance-free)—you either have to make your own or find a source for lotion made without artificial fragrances and all sorts of additives. We wonder why our body products are so saturated when many people have sensitivities and allergies to these substances.

Menstruums are liquids used to extract active constituents in plants and get them into solution so that they can be used. Water, vinegar, ethyl alcohol, glycerin and fixed oils are the menstruums available to the average person.

Neat's-foot oil is made from the feet and shin bones of cattle. Neat" is an archaic name for domestic bovine. This oil is used to waterproof leather goods and is sold as "neatsfoot oil".

Oils (Fixed) We buy small quantities of high quality seed oils for making herbal products. Oils become rancid because of oxidation without artificial preservative. There is no sense in wasting good money on large bottles that cannot be used quickly enough. Oils should be cold or expeller-pressed, preferably organic; you shouldn't put any oil *on* your skin that you wouldn't put *in* your body. We like to have a selection on hand.

Coconut oil is also called coconut butter. Cold-pressed, unrefined coconut butter is high in saturated fats which makes it stable when heated to high temperatures. It contains the anti-bacterial and anti-viral compound, lauric acid that is found in human breast milk. **Coconut oil** is very fatty—it is lubricating, not moisturizing—it is great for dry skin, but not for oily skin. Store at room temperature in a cool place, out of direct light.
Grape seed, according to Rebecca Woods, in *The New Whole Foods Encyclopedia*, we should restrict our use of grape seed oil

to that expressed from organically grown grapes. Chemical toxins concentrate in the fatty acids of plants.

Jojoba beans are pressed to extract their oil, producing a fine-quality oil used in skincare products. It is rich and expensive. No more than 10 % jojoba oil should be used in the total volume of a formula. Oils for human consumption (sometimes referred to as "fixed oils") are best when cold pressed and unprocessed. **Olive oil, almond oil** or **walnut oil** can be used to make ointments. If the oil is to be heated, olive oil or coconut butter is the best choice. Heating nut oils destroys beneficial fatty acids.
Massage-quality oils such as **almond, walnut, olive, sesame** or **grape seed** are cold pressed and good for the skin.
Vitamin E oil, in the form of **wheat germ oil**, should be added to oil preparations at a rate of 5 to 10 % of the total volume to help prevent or slow rancidity; it has a strong odor and a dark color. We keep it in the fridge for a longer shelf-life.

Shea butter is extracted from the nut kernel of the African shea nut bush (*Vitellaria paradoxa*). The fruits are collected from the ground around the trees and washed to remove soil and mold. The nuts are separated from the pulp, dried and then shelled. The seed is roasted and then ground into a powder. The oil is expressed either by cold- press extraction (preferred) or by hexane or other chemical means. Cold-expressed, food-grade shea butter is used in the manufacture of chocolates, cooking oil and in cosmetic lotions and creams.

Surfactants are substances that lower the surface tension of water. Many different types of surfactants are available online from sources providing herbal and cosmetic supplies (see our **sources**.) We are learning more about using different surfactants. Tina uses Shaklee® Basic H®, which is formulated with linear alcohol alkoxylates. This is the only ingredient listed on the label. It is found on the back panel under "Precautions & First Aid". The only precaution is to avoid contact with eyes. The company provides this information: Basic-H is pH neutral, non-irritating to skin and is concentrated. It is a low-sudsing and effective cleaner with no fragrance added. The company is not forthcoming when asked for further details. Except for the outlet in Tina's neighborhood of Mountain View, Arkansas, our shopping experiences with Shaklee have been limited, since the products are not available in stores.

In our search to find a reasonable facsimile, a surfactant without added fragrance, we found www.theherbsplace.com. These folks sell a surfactant called Sunshine Concentrate. It, too, contains linear alcohol alkoxylates, water and a substance listed as "Delaire DL", a mild, non-irritating fragrance. There is mention of a proprietary secret ingredient in the Sunshine product. Both companies use a "green" marketing message. However, we object to the difficulty we encounter trying to find out how these products are manufactured. Susan uses Dr. Bronner's Sal Suds, which is a blend of plant-based surfactants for all-purpose cleaning applications.

Sugar has fine grains, that, when combined with good quality oils, gently exfoliates old, dead cells from the skin. Sucrose is a water binding agent, that is, it helps the skin retain moisture. *Be gentle with your skin and don't overuse any exfoliant. Skin can become photosensitized and irritated.*

Vinegar can be apple cider or distilled for external use. For best health benefits for internal use, raw apple cider or grape vinegar is preferred. Raw, unpasteurized apple cider vinegar is 6% acidity. Acidity in vinegar preserves plant material and is antibacterial. (see **washing greens** in **household preparations** for a report

on vinegar and *E. coli)* Raw apple cider vinegar contributes 50
nutrients, amino acids and trace elements to the value of the
preparation.

Vinegar is antiseptic and healing to the skin. Commercial vinegar
is diluted with water to approximately 5% acidity. Some folks need
to dilute it further before using it on the skin or scalp.

Homemade vinegar should not be used unless the acid level is
between 4 to 6 percent and it has been pasteurized. Vinegar owes
its preservative qualities to the mild acetic acid content. Do not add
water to flavored vinegars, as this would dilute the acid. Be sure
to cover the herb completely with vinegar to avoid the growth of
mold. Discard any moldy vinegar. Vinegar that develops a mother
or becomes ropy and cloudy can be strained, brought to a boil and
rebottled. Store vinegars, tightly capped, in a cool dark place.

We do not use distilled vinegar, except for cleaning house. Rebecca
Wood, author of *The New Whole Foods Encyclopedia*, in reference
to distilled vinegar states, "By FDA regulations since the 1950s,
it may be synthetic ethanol made by direct chemical oxidation of
wood or fossil fuels. Distilled and other highly processed vinegars
are mineral deficient, and when consumed, pull calcium and other
minerals from the bones and tissues".

For more information on making vinegars for culinary use, see our
chapter on **infusions & decoctions**.

Water quality is an important concern in making herbal products.
Choose distilled water, clear soft water or purified rainwater. Hard
water contains minerals, such as lime, which foster precipitation.
Distilled water is used to make spritzers and to dilute alcohol when
making tinctures. Water has no ability to preserve the herbs. Water

does not extract alcohol solvent materials. Water does provide an effective medium for getting herbal infusions, decoctions and fomentations to a sick or injured person.

Witch hazel astringent is the inner bark of *Hamamelis virginiana* tinctured in ethanol content of 70 to 80 percent. It can be drying to the skin because of the high alcohol content. The herb is very high in tannins, which are antioxidants that harden and heal the proteins in skin. If it is used repeatedly, witch hazel astringent can be irritating.

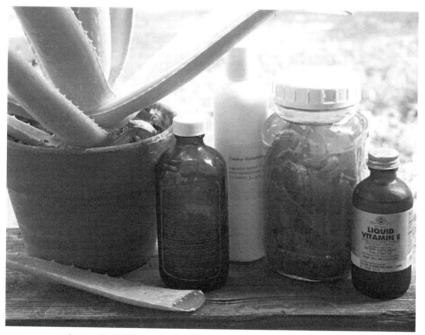

aloe, distillates, vinegar and vitamin E oil are ingredients in our herbal pantry

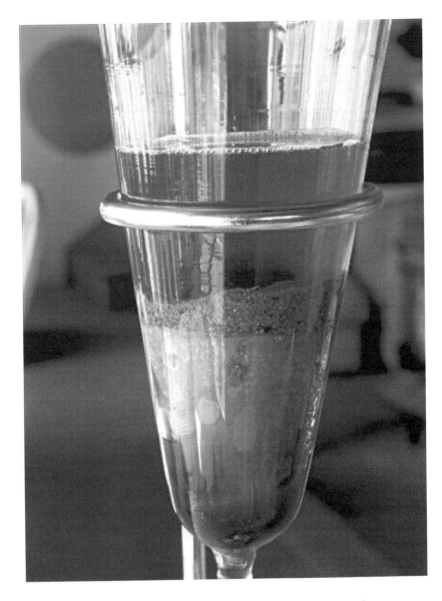

*percolation cone with alcohol menstruum for
making tinctures*

definition of terms

The goal of this section is to shed the light of understanding on words commonly found in herbals. The more one knows and understands, the more benefit can be gained. We encourage you to become familiar with these terms, as well as the herbs that you use.

alkaloids—are alkaline compounds that contain nitrogen and have potent effects on the circulatory and nervous systems of the body.

allergen—a substance that causes an allergic reaction.

analgesic—a substance or remedy that relieves pain.

anesthetic—loss of sensation; or an agent that causes the absence of feeling.

anti-bacterial—kills or inhibits the growth of bacteria.

antibiotic—prevents the growth of, or destroys microorganisms such as bacteria.

antidepressant—aids in preventing and relieving depression.

anti-fungal—helps prevent and destroy fungus.

anti-inflammatory—reduces inflammation (although some inflammation may be necessary for healing).

anti-microbial—destroys and prevents the production of pathogenic microorganisms (anti-bacterial and anti-viral).

antioxidant—helps the body fight free radicals, by delaying oxidation or deterioration, particularly when exposed to air.

anti-putrescent—a substance that inhibits putrefaction and fights decay.

antiseptic— a substance that stops sepsis which is the infectious breakdown of body tissue; destroys and prevents the growth of microorganisms.

anti-spasmodic—eases or prevents spasms and cramping.

antitoxin—an antidote to counteract the effects of a poisonous substance.

anti-venomous—an agent that is an antitoxin to venom.

anti-viral—prevents the proliferation or inhibits growth of viruses.

aphrodisiac—a substance that increases and excites sexual desire.

astringent—causes contraction and firming of organic tissues, which decreases the amount of body secretions and discharge.

bactericidal—destroys or inhibits the growth of bacteria.

bioflavonoid—a plant glycoside that is diuretic, anti-spasmodic, anti-inflammatory and improves circulation.

carminative—helps to stimulate the digestive tract, soothe the stomach and relieve flatulence.

carrier—can be distilled water, vinegar, alcohol, surfactants, soap, baking soda and corn starch, oil or a bit of material to which essential oils are added to diffuse them for use.

carrier oil—a base oil from plant seeds or nuts, usually used with essential oils to dilute them, since most EOs cannot be applied directly (neat) to the skin.

cathartic—synonymous with purgative , a strong, rapidly acting laxative used to relieve severe constipation.

compress—also called a fomentation, it is applied to inflamed, cold or congested areas of the body. Sprains, strained muscles, boils and congestion may be helped with this activity. Choose the appropriate therapeutic herb and make an infusion with it. Submerge a clean, absorbent cloth in the infusion. With a pair of tongs, pull the cloth out and let it cool until you can squeeze out the excess infusion. Place the warm, steaming cloth on an injury or wound. Cover with a larger towel to hold in the heat. Leave in place for about 30 minutes. Use cold compresses for hot inflammations or alternate between cold and hot.

concentrates—are made by simmering an infusion or decoction to reduce the volume of water by more than half the amount or more.

decoction—an herbal preparation made from the hard or woody parts of plants by boiling them in water to concentrate their healing virtues; see the chapter on infusions and decoctions.

demulcent—a soothing substance that protects mucous membranes and prevents irritation.

deodorant—a substance that changes, covers, or removes disagreeable odors.

diaphoretic—increases perspiration and cleansing through the skin.

digestive—an agent that aids or promotes digestion.

distillate—the result of the steam distillation of fragrant plants to remove essential oils; hydrosol is another name for this mildly aromatic liquid that is left once the EO has been extracted.

diuretic—a substance that stimulates the elimination of body wastes through the kidney and bladder.

emetic—a substance that induces vomiting.

emollient—soothes, softens and protects inflamed tissues.

essential oils—these concentrated EOs are made from fragrant plant materials, usually prepared by steam distillation, sometimes with CO_2; they are very strong essences and should be used carefully and sparingly. See our chapter on essential oils.

estrogenic—is a substance that stimulates female hormonal activity. expectorant—assists the respiratory system by helping to remove excess mucus from the lungs.

extracts—are infusions, decoctions, vinegars or tinctures.

floral water—(or flower water) is different from a hydrosol or distillate since it is not made from a steam distillation; they are usually prepared by adding fragrant oils (most common are rose, orange and violet) to distilled water. They can be prepared by simmering flowers in water, discarding the spent flowers and adding fresh ones repeatedly until the water becomes tinted and fragrant.

fomentation—(synonymous with compress), is usually prepared by making an herbal infusion (can be other liquids like oil or just hot water) and applying it to the body or wounded area with hot cloths that have been steeped in the infusion. At least two cloths are necessary to keep them continually hot—cotton flannel or wool is best for this sort of compress. A sheet of plastic can be used to hold in moisture and temperature. Cold fomentations are used for sprains and to stop bleeding. A water bag, filled with hot or cold water can be added to maintain the appropriate temperature and add comforting weight. Alternating cold and hot fomentations may be appropriate.

fungicidal—inhibits the growth of fungi.

furocoumarins, or **furanocoumarins**, are present in citrus oils, citrus peels, fig sap, rue and some composite family plants. The skin is exposed to the oils of these plants through application of homemade insect repellents or fragrances; by squeezing limes, oranges or lemons for their juice; applying tanning lotions and creams; and working with plants that contain furocoumarins. When the skin is simultaneously exposed to sunlight or tanning lights, (UVA radiation) an allergic reaction occurs that is called phototoxicity. The furocoumarins absorb the energy of photons and releases it into skin cells, causing damage to the DNA. For more information, see **plant chemicals**.

glycerin — is a triatomic alcohol and the sweet principle of oils.

hydrosol — see distillate.

hypnotic — relaxes and sedates; induces sleep (does not cause hypnotic trance).

infusion — the steeping or infusing of herb leaves or flowers, usually in water, in order to extract their virtues; see the chapter on infusions and decoctions.

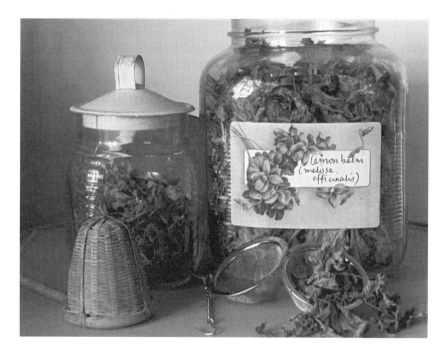

lemon balm is one of our favorite herbal infusions and has sedative properties

insecticidal—a substance that kills insects.

larvicidal— is a substance used to kill larval pests.

maceration—to macerate, infuse, or steep plant material in a solvent (menstruum such as water, alcohol, vinegar, etc.) until the material is soft or digested or mixture (such as fruit salad) to extract its virtues or flavor.

marc—the solid material that is left after the menstruum (liquid) has been removed as in making a tincture. The word is derived from the French *marcher* meaning to trample, thus marc also refers to the residue that is left after pressing grapes or apples for juice.

menstruum—this is the solvent or liquid that is used in extracting the virtues from herbs as in making a tincture; it can be all or parts water, alcohol, glycerin, vinegar, or wine. Different menstruums work better with different herbs—the idea is to find the best solution to extract the constituents that you desire—and leave the ones that you don't want. This takes practice being an herbalist or reading from herb books.

microbe—is microscopic organism, such as bacteria, fungi and viruses.

mortar and pestle—an ancient tool and a must-have piece of equipment for grinding herbs and seeds, and making poultices; the mortar and pestle was truly the first tool used to make medicine. The Italian verb *pestare* means to pound, crush, tread or beat. The mortar is the bowl-shaped container and the pestle is the rod-shaped device with a rounded end, which is used for pounding or grinding whatever is in the mortar. We recommend a high-fired vitrous porcelain or stone mortar and pestle, rather than a wooden one.

mucilaginous—a substance having demulcent, gelatinous qualities; soothes inflammation.

neat—this term is used by aromatherapists and herbalists when referring to applying an essential oil directly on the skin, undiluted. This is not recommended, with the exception of a very few EOs; please see our chapter on essential oils for more information.

nervine—an agent that relaxes, tones or stimulates the nervous system, depending upon the attributes of the chosen herb.

parasiticidal—a substance that helps to destroy parasites such as fleas and lice.

patch test—people have different sensitivities to plants and oils. If you have very sensitive skin or are taking prescription medication, it is prudent to do a "patch test" for every new essential oil before exposing larger areas of your body to the oil. Mix three drops of the essential oil to 1/2 teaspoon carrier oil. Apply this mixture to the pad of a Band-Aid® and secure the bandage to the inner part of the forearm. Leave on for 48 hours. If the area shows any irritation under or around the patch, the EO should not be used. Also see skin test. *Caution: Pregnant and nursing women and those who suffer from plant allergies should consult with their health care providers before using essential oils and herbs.*

pathogenic—disease producing.

percolation—the act of preparing a tincture in a percolation cone rather than as an infusion; it is much more expedient with an end result in as few as two days. For more information see tinctures chapter.

phototoxic—certain substances have a damaging toxic effect when triggered by exposing the skin to light; this is especially common with the citrus essential oils—so keep this in mind when using them—read your labels.

poultice—a preparation made from fresh herbs or powdered plant material that is made into a paste with hot water; they are usually applied to a cloth and placed directly on the body. Poultices need to be kept hot, so the application of a piece of plastic and a heating pad or hot water bottle helps to facilitate holding moist heat in; otherwise the poultice needs to be changed as it cools. Dried plant materials are moistened with water or vinegar. Fresh materials are pounded, chopped, mashed, or chewed and placed directly on the body. Poultices should be applied thick and wet but not runny. If the poultice is applied warm, do not reheat and reuse.

precipitate—means to separate and settle. Precipitate substances can be floating in a solution or settle down to the bottom of the container, forming a deposit of solid matter. Precipitates are formed in a solution by the action of chemical agents or certain physical forces, such as low temperature. See the chapter on tinctures for further details.

prophylactic—protects against infection and disease. restorative—a substance that aids in strengthening and revitalizing the body and mind.

sedative—a substance that reduces stress, calms the nervous system and helps to relax the body.

shrub—an old-fashioned beverage made from alcoholic liquor or vinegar; fruit, fruit juice and/or rind; and sugar. These are aged in crockery or glass, and then poured off and served alone, or with sparkling or seltzer water over ice. They are very refreshing and often cause perspiration; see our recipe for shrub.

simple—this is an old term used for making a medicinal preparation having only one ingredient; a plant used for its supposed medicinal properties.

skin test—is a quick and less scientific way to test a substance on your skin instead of a patch test. Always test for individual allergic reactions to homemade substances before applying them to large areas of the body. A simple skin test is to drop a little of the concoction on the inner arm (elbow crease is convenient) and wait 30 to 60 minutes, especially if you have allergies or sensitive skin. If the skin does not redden or blister, you should be good to go.

soporific—sleep-inducing substance.

spritzer—sometimes called a mister, these aromatherapy products are made from distilled water and essential oils; when spritzed they can relax and calm or stimulate depending upon the EOs that are used. See recipes for various mood-elevating spritzers in our body care chapter.
stimulant—a substance that speeds up body functions, as well as the mind.

surfactant—a soap or a detergent, which is able to solublize both water and oil thus allowing them to mix. The molecule itself has two ends—one that is the water soluble end—and one that is the oil soluble end. These are used to make cleaning products for the home as well as in cosmetics (see definition of terms).

syrup—is made with sugar or honey—at a proportion of 2 parts sugar/honey to 1 part water—which preserves the herbal extract. Syrup has the advantage of being sticky which helps the medicinal adhere to tissues longer than straight liquid. Syrup is the usual menstruum for cough remedies; "Just a spoonful of sugar helps the medicine go down." However, sometimes a sick person may not be able to tolerate the sweet flavor.

tincture—prepared by infusion or percolation, a tincture is made from herbs—root, leaf, stem and/or flower—from fresh or dried plant material. A menstruum or solvent such as diluted alcohol, glycerin or vinegar is used to extract the attributes of the herbs. Please see our chapter on tinctures for more information.

tonic—certain agents used to tonify specific parts or the whole body, providing vitality and strength to tissues and body systems.

triturate—is to pulverize or grind to a fine powder.

vermifuge—destroys and expels worms.

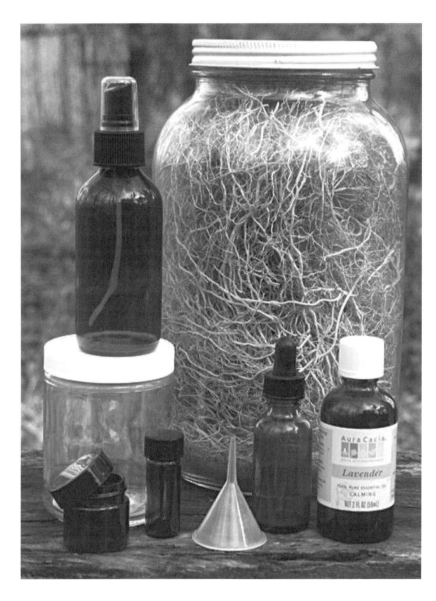

our sources will help you find bottles, jars, dried herbs, oils, ingredients and equipment

sources

There are many herbal resources out there—we can't begin to mention all of them—here are some that we have satisfactorily used. We cannot be held accountable for your transactions.

American Herbalists Guild www.americanherbalist.com
1931 Gaddis Road
Canton, GA 30115
professional organization for herb practitioners; great sourcebook

American College of Health Care Studies www.achs.edu
accredited courses in herbalism and aromatherapy; complete apothecary shop sells EOs, dried herbs, equipment, and more

Desert Bloom Herbs www.desertbloomherbs.com
1606 North Florida
Silver City, NM 88061
bulk herbs, herbal products, percolation cone kit

Frontier Herbs www.frontiercoop.com
3021 78th Street
Norway, IA 52318
well-known source for dried herbs, EOs, oils, and more

International Herb Association www.iherb.org
PO Box 5667
Jacksonville, FL 32247
herb business organization; annual booklet on Herb of the Year

Healing Hollers www.healin-hollers.com
handcrafted herbal products; Diggers' Guide to Medicinal Plants

Healing Spirits www.healingspirits.com
9198 Route 415
Avoca, NY 14809
good-quality wildcrafted and organically grown herbs

Heartsong Farm Healing Herbs www.herbsandapples.com
Nancy and Michael Phillips
RFD 1 Box 275 Lost Nation Road
Groveton, NH 03582
excellent-quality organic dried herbs, handcrafted tinctures, homemade apple cider vinegar; The Village Herbalist

Herb Companion www.herbcompanion.com

Herb Growing & Marketing Network www.herbworld.com
PO Box 245
Silver Spring, PA 17575
great source for herbal info; Herbalpedia cd

Herb Society of America www.herbsociety.org
9019 Kirtland Chardon Road
Kirtland, OH 44094
nation's oldest herbal organization has informative web site with herb of the year info; publishes The Herbarist annually

HerbalGram www.herbalgram.org, Journal of the American Botanical Council

The Herbarie www.theherbarie.com
excellent source for info, herbs, oils, surfactants and much more

Herbs for Health www.herbsforhealth.com
Mountain Rose Herbals www.mountainroseherbs.com
85472 Dilley Lane
Eugene, OR 97405
great source for dried herbs, EOs, and every sort of herbal need

Sage Mountain Herbal Retreat Center & Botanical Sanctuary
Rosemary Gladstar www.sagemountain.com
PO Box 420
East Barre, VT 05649
Rosemary's books; Science and Art of Herbalism course

Sagescript Institute, LLC www.sagescript.com
Cindy Jones
wonderful distillates, herb products, informative books, and more

SKS Bottles www.sks-bottle.com
great source for any kind of bottle, jar, vial, and equipment

Rich Gulch Products www.mathrespresses.com
tincture press

United Plant Savers www.unitedplantsavers.org
PO Box 98
East Barre, VT 05649
non-profit group dedicated to protecting native medicinal plants

Zack Woods Herb Farm zackwoods@pshift.com
278 Mead Road
Hyde Park, VT 05655
excellent-quality organic dried herbs

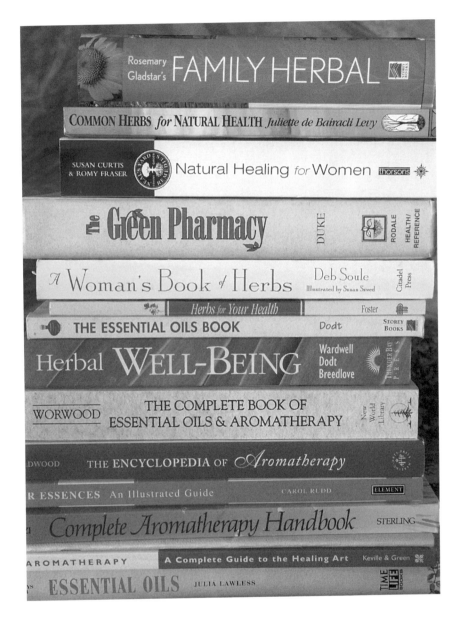

some books in our herbal library

bibliography

Asimov, Isaac. *The World of Carbon*. New York: Collier Books, 1979.

Balch, Phyllis A., CNC. *Prescription for Herbal Healing*. New York: Avery Publishing, 2002.

Belsinger, Susan. 2007. Meeting healing head-on with herbs. *Herb Companion* Vol. 19 No. 2: 40-45.

_____. 2006. See you later, alligator: say goodbye to dry skin. *Herb Companion* Vol. 19, No. 1:15-19.

Blumgarten, AS, M.D., F.A.C.P. *Textbook of Materia Medica*. New York: Macmillan Company, 1925.

Bown, Deni. *Encyclopedia of Herbs and Their Uses*. New York: Dorling Kindersley, 1995.

Chevallier, Andrew. *The Encyclopedia of Medicinal Plants*. New York: Dorling Kindersley, 1996.

Dodt, Colleen K. *The Essential Oils Book*. North Adams, Massachusetts: Storey Books, 1996.

Duke, James A., Ph.D. *Herb-A-Day*. Virginia Beach: Eco Images, 2007.

_____. *The Green Pharmacy*. Emmaus, Pennsylvania: Rodale Press, 1997.

Fischer-Rizzi, Susan. *Complete Aromatherapy Handbook*. New York: Sterling Publishing Company, 1990.

Foley, Daniel J. *Herbs for Use and Delight*. New York: Dover Publications, 1974.

Foster, Steven, and Duke, James A. *A Field Guide to Medicinal Plants: Eastern and Central North America*. Boston: Houghton Mifflin Company, 1990.

Foster, Steven, and Johnston, Rebecca L. *National Geographic Desk Reference to Nature's Medicine*. Washington, D.C.: National Geographic, 2006

Foster, Steven, and Tyler, Varro E. *Tyler's Honest Herbal*. Binghamton, New York: Haworth Herbal Press, 1998.

Gladstar, Rosemary. *Rosemary Gladstar's Family Herbal*. North Adams, Massachusetts: Storey Books, 2001.

Green, James. *The Herbal Medicine Maker's Handbook: a Home Manual*. Freedom, California: The Crossing Press, 2000.

Grieve, Maud. *A Modern Herbal*. New York: Dover Publications, 1982.

Hoffman, David. *The Herbal Handbook: A User's Guide to Medical Herbalism*. Rochester, Vermont: Healing Arts Press, 1988.

Hunter, Carl. *Trees, Shrubs & Vines of Arkansas*. Little Rock: The Ozark Society Foundation, 1995.

Hylton, William H., editor. *The Rodale Herb Book*. Emmaus, Pennsylvania: Rodale Press, 1979.

Keville, Kathi, and Green, Mindi. *Aromatherapy: A Complete Guide to the Healing Art*. Freedom, California: The Crossing Press, 1995.

Lawless, Julia. *Natural Ways to Health with Essential Oils*. Alexandria, Virginia: Time-Life Books, 1995.

Miles, Karen. *Herb & Spice Handbook*. Norway, Iowa: Frontier Cooperative Herbs, 1987.

Moore, Michael. *Medicinal Plants of the Desert and Canyon West*. Santa Fe: Museum of New Mexico Press, 1989.

Phillips, Nancy and Michael. *The Village Herbalist*. White River Junction, Vermont: Chelsea Green Publishing Company, 2001.

Rogers, Maureen. *Herbalpedia 2007*. Silver Spring, Pennsylvania: The Herb Growing & Marketing Network, 2007

Soule, Deb. *A Woman's Book of Herbs*. Secaucus, New Jersey, 1995.

Tierra, Michael, L.Ac., O.M.D. *The Way of Herbs*. New York: Pocket Books, 1998.

Tisserand, Robert and Balacs, Tony . *Essential Oil Safety: A Guide for Health Care Professionals*. Edinburgh: Churchill Livingstone, 1995.

Traunfeld, Jerry. *The Herbfarm Cookbook*. New York: Scribner, 2000.

Tucker, Arthur O. and DeBaggio, Thomas. *The Big Book of Herbs*. Loveland, Colorado: Interweave Press, 2000.

Walters, Clare. *Aromatherapy: An Illustrated Guide*. Boston: Element Books Limited, 1998.

Wilcox, Tina Marie, and Belsinger, Susan. 2006. Nix the Itch of Summer. *Herb Companion* July: 27-31.

_____. 2002. Echinacea: The Art of tincturing. *Herbs for Health* September: 24-28.

Wildwood, Chrissie. *The Encyclopedia of Aromatherapy*. Rochester, Vermont: Healing Arts Press, 1996.

Wood, Rebecca. *The New Whole Foods Encyclopedia*. New York: Penguin Books, 1999.

Worwood, Valerie Ann. *The Complete Book of Essential Oils and Aromatherapy*. San Rafael, California: New World Library, 1991.

web sites

Veterinarian topical therapy information.
http://acvdresidents.tripod.com/home/review/Pharmacology/
TOPICAL%20THERAY.doc

James A. Duke FDA list of GRAS (Generally Recognized as Safe)
list of herbs http://www.ars-grin.gov/duke/syllabus/gras.htm

Purdue Guide to Medicinal and Aromatic Plants: *Pennyroyal*
http://www.hort.purdue.edu/newcrop/med-aro/factsheets/
PENNYROYAL.html

Australian honey producers with articles on the health benefits
www.hythes.com

Sheabutter production and uses http://www.sekafghana.com/
sheabutter.html

University of Minnosota, *Essential Oil Safety*
http://takingcharge.csh.umn.edu/therapies/aromatherapy/are_
essential_oils_safe

The Internet Dermatology Society, Inc, *Phytophotodermatitis*
http://telemedicine.org/botanica/bot5.htm

Medline Plus: *Pennyroyal*
http://www.nlm.nih.gov/medlineplus/druginfo/natural/patient-
pennyroyal.html

Honey as a topical antibacterial for treatment of infected wounds.
http://www.worldwidewounds.com/2001/november/Molan/honey-
as-topical-agent.html#

index

chapter titles are in boldface; numbers in boldface are photos

notes

living with herbs

look for these titles in the series
published by herbspirit

the creative herbal home
susan belsinger & tina marie wilcox
publication date summer 2007

not just desserts — sweet herbal recipes
susan belsinger
published in 2005

the savory herbal
a collection of vegetarian recipes
susan belsinger
publication date fall 2011

the creative herbal garden
tina marie wilcox & susan belsinger
publication date spring 2012

to order these books:
for single retail copies or bulk wholesale

contact: susan belsinger
web site: www.susanbelsinger.com